I dedicate this book to my three sisters, Debbie, Terri, and Rhonda because we are all in this together!

Muscle-up
for
Menopause™

Published by MajorVision International

2021

Approved by The World Isometric Exercise Association

www.TWiEA.com

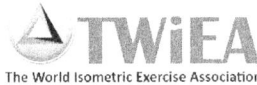

The World Isometric Exercise Association

WWW.MAJORVISION.COM

Contents

Important General Safety and Health Guidelines

This section pertains to The ISOfitness™ Exercise System and team, TWIEA (The World Isometric Exercise Association), any association, collaboration and partnership, any associated online resources, all print and e-books, courses, publications, articles, videos, associated websites, recommendations, suggestions, coaching, advice either written, cyber, or verbal that is given, implied, or suggested, all courses authored and/or delivered by Brian Sterling-Vete and Helen Renée Wuorio, the copyright holders, creators, writers, instructors, and the originators of the material including but not limited to The Bullworker 90™ Course, The Bullworker Bible™, The Bullworker Compendium™, The Doorway to Strength™, Feel Better in 70-Seconds™, Fitness on the Move™, Isometric Exercises for Nordic Walking and Trekking Pt 1 & 2, Improvised Isometric Exercise Devices (IIED) The Climber's Sling™, Improvised Isometric Exercise Devices (IIED) The Daisy Chain™, Isometric Power Exercises for Martial Artists™, The ISO90™ Course, Isometric Exercises for Golf Pt 1 & 2, The ISOmetric Bible™, Muscle Up for Menopause™, The Sixty Second Ass Workout™, The 70 Second Difference™, The TRISO90™ Course, TRISOmetrics™, The Zero Footprint Lockdown Workout™, and The Workout at Work™. You should never begin any kind of sport, exercise system, workout plan, or diet modification, including everything contained in this book and in any books mentioned in the beginning paragraph above unless you have consulted with and have the full approval of your medical doctor.

Your physician can accurately assess your current health status, and your ability to perform the exercises in the book and/or course. This is particularly important if you have any known or unknown pre-existing health issues, if you are pregnant, or if you believe that you may have other serious health conditions.

You must always have absolute approval from your physician before starting. Please show all the material in the above courses, books, video/audio, online material, and all other content to your physician to get their approval before you start.

All exercises, suggestions, recommendations, instructions, exercise plans, dietary and eating recommendations, either given or implied or anything that falls under paragraph 1 is only intended as a reference source, and it is no substitute for a qualified professional personal coach to plan an exercise and diet program appropriate for your age and physical condition. Also, nothing mentioned in paragraph 1 is intended for use by children, and all exercise equipment must be kept out of their reach.

Never overexert yourself when performing any exercise. Stop exercising immediately and consult your doctor if you ever experience any pain, irregular heartbeat, shortness of breath, tightness in your chest/arms/fingers, faintness, nausea, or feelings of dizziness. Then consult your doctor and/or call the EMS immediately.

Always inspect any exercise equipment, and/or any/all other improvised or specifically made exercise equipment/materials, doors, door jambs, and door frames, and anything else you use before each use to ensure its proper operation and to ensure that it is undamaged and safe. Do not use it unless all parts are free from wear, and it is functioning properly. To avoid serious injury, care should always be taken using any/all exercise equipment, and in all items, people, books, and courses mentioned in paragraph 1 of this section. Care should always be taken when getting into all exercise positions, on and off the floor, on and off chairs, on and off benches, on and off any other surface that might be used for exercise, including pieces of furniture, and in the use of all exercised equipment, either purpose-made or improvised.

No person, people, team, company, or organisation mentioned in paragraph 1 of this section can accept any responsibility whatsoever for any injury, harm, damage, illness, harm, damage to property, or any other negative health-related condition which may occur as a direct, or indirect result of following these courses, recommendations, suggestions, diagrams, pictures, videos, or while performing any exercises in these or any related other related material/publication/s.

For additional general information, we also recommend that you check reputable accredited medical advice sites such as The National Health Service in the United Kingdom, online at: https://www.nhs.uk/Livewell/fitness/pages/physical-activity-guidelines-for-adults.aspx

And: https://www.mayoclinic.org/healthy-lifestyle

Chapter 1: Preface

I am no celebrity, I am just an ordinary person, as is my husband. However, he is a world-leading authority on all forms of isometric and TRISOmetric™ exercise. Also, I have now been highly trained in the science of exercise by my husband and from other sources. Unfortunately, despite all of this, many people will never read this book because it was not 'written' by some sort of celebrity.

Some people seem to believe that TV and media celebrities somehow gain some miraculous influx because of nothing else except their celebrity status. Therefore, if a celebrity puts their name to a book about exercise, then surely, they must know all that there is to know about the subject – right?

Wrong... Almost always, celebrities who put their name to such books have had a team of fitness experts and ghost writers research and prepare the book for them so they can approve it and put their name to it. Also, the celebrity in question typically knows little or nothing about the subject other than what their research team or personal trainer has told them. This is simply part of the culture we live in today.

Why am I making these points? I do so to highlight the fact that one does not need to be a media celebrity to know about exercise and nutrition. Nor do you need to be a celebrity to be able to produce a valuable resource about how diet and exercise can help significantly as you navigate your way through menopause.

My journey into and through menopause is real and I am about three-quarters of the way through it, or perhaps a little more to date as I write this book. Therefore, my story is gritty, soul-bearing, often embarrassing, and I sincerely hope that some may even find it both inspirational and helpful. More importantly, when it comes to dealing with menopause in general and many of the common problems that almost everyone will face, we offer simple solutions that are practical, scientifically proven, inexpensive, achievable, and functional.

The fact is that almost everyone can do these things if they want to minimise the impact of menopause badly enough and manage their journey through it. Make no mistake, menopause can be a challenge for anyone, but with the right proactive approach, it makes life a whole lot easier and much more pleasant. Therefore, we hope that you find the practical advice in the contents of this book useful and life-enhancing as you navigate your unique way through menopause.

Chapter 2: Helen's Story

My name is Helen Renée Wuorio and I was born in Duluth Minnesota, in 1970, but as I write these words as I am sitting in our home in Manchester, England happily married to a British gentleman I adore. However, even though my new husband and I now live almost the entire year in England, we still keep a small pied-à-terre in Minnesota for when we revisit my native land. So, we get the best of both worlds in many respects, especially when it comes to enjoying four distinct seasons.

To get to England and this point in life has been, a remarkable journey, some of which I will share with you now because it will give you a more complete background to this book, the suggestions I offer, and the points that I make. Even though I am originally from the American Midwest, I am quite certain that almost all women will be able to relate to some of what I have been through in my life. In short, I know that I am not alone in my experiences, and I am not special, far from it because all women face the same biological journey and challenges. However, some of the practical solutions I found, together with what I have learned through a combination of trial and error, and painstaking research, might be useful for others who are either facing or going through similar life challenges.

My identical twin sister and I enjoyed a very happy childhood, and we shared many wonderful adventures with our parents. Perhaps the most exciting and remarkable life adventure during this formative time in our lives was when my father became an ice road trucker and we suddenly upped sticks and moved as a family to the land of the midnight sun, Alaska. When I think about it at this point in my life, I still get a huge kick out of the fact that our names, as a family, are listed in an engraving on the memorial shrine as being Pioneers of Fairbanks Alaska!

As a teenager, one of my passions at school was gymnastics, and I became quite good at this discipline because I had a petite but well-balanced, generally athletic build with a good power-to-weight muscle ratio. Other than that, I would participate in all the usual sports taught in the high schools of the day. These were probably little or no difference to the type of sports and activities most girls in western countries participate in. Except, perhaps, for compulsory dogsledding classes. Many people reading this would be forgiven for doing a double-take to read the previous sentence again, and then perhaps even giggle a little and find this part of our high school curriculum a little hard to comprehend. However, those would be people who either rarely or have never experienced truly deep snow each year and temperatures that drop way below zero for months at a time. Even people who live in places that get four seasons each year typically have only the vaguest idea about the severity of Alaskan cold and snow. To give you a better indication of how brutal it can be, on my school prom night it was 90 degrees Fahrenheit below zero wind chill. In fact, it was so cold that when a classmate slammed their car door shut it snapped off and fell to the ground.

As I grew, for me at least, I naturally became interested in boys and began to date. Eventually, after kissing a few metaphorical frogs along the way, I found a Prince Charming and very soon found myself happily married at the age of twenty-one and setting up my first home back in my native Minnesota. For many years we were blissfully happy, and I gave birth to two wonderful children three years apart, a boy and a girl. However, as the children grew, and as life generally progressed, I began to feel that I needed more from life, and more importantly, more than what I was getting from the relationship with my current husband. Perhaps it was some sort of early mid-life glitch, or perhaps it was for other reasons, I will never know for certain because looking back now it is such a grey and fuzzy area for me. However, the fact was that we simply grew apart over the years because we shared different views and ambitions about what each of us wanted out of life.

The upshot of it all was that even though the children were 11 and 14 years old respectively by this time, I filed for a divorce and we began working towards some sort of amicable and practical parenting solutions. Fortunately, my now ex-husband was and still is, a reasonable person, so we soon agreed upon a sensible and functional plan.

With the divorce papers eventually signed, sealed, and delivered, this was the start of a brave new world for me in every respect. I knew that things would now never be the same as my previously warm and cosy tater-tot hotdish former type of life, however, I was still vibrantly optimistic about embracing every aspect of what my new future held. I should add that tater-tot hotdish is a famous Minnesotan recipe synonymous with all the comforting feel-good things about life and people who come from the Midwest.)

As a newly divorced woman with children who were old enough to be left alone for a while, the first thing I did was get a decent job with a big company located near the city of Minneapolis. This was not as easy as it sounds. To get a job was actually a full-time job in and of itself due to the masses of paperwork involved that was always different for each company. It took me nearly a year of filing literally hundreds of job applications either directly or through employment agencies until I was accepted by a company I respected and in a capacity that challenged me and yet I still found comfortable.

To this day, I often marvel at the people in human resources. This is because two of the jobs I applied for were with companies I had worked for previously in the same role. I had not only excelled in the role, but I had also won significant awards for doing the job. In addition, my application had the full backing of the immediate senior management who knew me well and were not only happy to learn that I wanted to return they were also extremely supportive and keen to help me get the job. What happened? I did not even receive an interview offer for either job opportunity.

During my time as a professional job seeker writing out long laborious job applications, when I was not a full-time mother of two fast-growing teenagers, I was either temping through agencies or performing menial jobs here, there, and everywhere just to scrape a living. I was certainly doing nothing whatsoever to take care of myself physically, or emotionally. Therefore, my once youthful and to a degree formerly natural athletic look I had previously somehow maintained was fast becoming a long-forgotten memory of my late teens and early twenties. Leading a comfortable life before marriage, having two children, and now the ever more onerous time-consuming responsibilities divorce brings with it in its wake, were taking their toll on me physically and beginning to wreak havoc with my health.

Thankfully, I eventually found myself in quite a senior executive role in a wonderful new job. This meant that in general, life became much more structured and predictable again, and far more comfortable due to the substantial salary I earned. In short, life became good again! instead of disciplining myself to perform even just the most basic regular exercise routine, I did nothing. The closest thing to strength training that I was performing was using all the strength I could muster to pull the cork out of several bottles of red wine each evening as I relaxed after work. In addition, it was all too easy to either order takeaway or eat out, so on reflection, my diet was appallingly bad. This was my new normal, and soon my petite 4 feet 11 inches formerly athletic frame began to alarmingly resemble the Michelin Man figure I would see on the side of trucks. I was a fatty, there is no other way to describe myself. Also, there is no way to dress it up and say I felt 'comfortable' with my body, just the way I was. This would have been a lie, because I did not feel comfortable, and I was anything but healthy.

Was I motivated enough to do anything about it? No, not at all. Part of the problem was that even though I knew that I was a fatty, I could still look quite good in clothes and hide it well. By simply choosing the right things to wear meant that I could usually get away with the physical manifestations of my appalling lifestyle choices, which had sadly become the new normal for me.

Since I could still look good in clothes despite hiding a few bulges here and there. Also, by general standards, I was more or less normal as far as most women of that age go. It was not too long before I started to explore dating again. So, I signed up to some of the better dating sites to see who was out there, and to my surprise, I was soon inundated with offers of all kinds. Perhaps what surprised me the most, was that I had dozens of offers from men in their early to mid-twenties. I knew full-well that they were only interested in one thing, this was the older attractive woman experience.

Did I care? Not one iota. I had an almost constant choice of some really attractive young studs, all with fabulous, hard, muscular, and attractive bodies. Life was good, and I do not care if my honesty and openness about it all surprises or offends anybody reading this. Besides, who are they to judge me? Did I receive any emotional fulfilment from all these young guys? Did I have any deep and meaningful conversations about life, love, spirituality, the human condition, and the universe in general? No, nothing whatsoever, it was all about sex for me.

Eventually, the magic of the young studs began to wane, and I began to look for more in a man. In truth, I realised that I was ready for a proper relationship again. I felt in my heart that the time was right in my life to seek out a man who would be my end-game life mate, a partner who I would be with for the rest of my life. I do not know if it was fate, or in hindsight black magic, but it was not too long before I was introduced by friends to the one, the man of my dreams. He was amazing in every respect and to add even more sparkle to it all, he was foreign, from a very wealthy family in Gabon and he was in the USA as a post-graduate student. This amazing man was charming, polite, and attentive. Furthermore, he was savagely handsome, muscular, tall, dark-skinned, and with a striking dark-eyed face that was almost feminine in his masculine beauty. The result? It was not long before we were married, and I was leading a lifestyle involving lots of international travel back and forth across the globe.

For me, someone who in their mind's eye, was just an average girl from the Midwest, this was a dream come true. And yet on reflection, this man somehow possessed a world-weary air of either someone much older than his years or someone harbouring dark secrets. If only it had been the former, but sadly, it was the latter that turned out to be true.

And as the light of truth shone ever more brightly upon him, layer by layer it revealed something disconcertingly serpent-like in his increasingly aloof appearance and demeanour. The dream marriage to my dream man soon became the worst nightmare imaginable...

2014 is a year that will be indelibly graven upon my recollection. Why? Because at 44 years of age I suddenly found myself single again. My dream man from Gabon had become the cause of incalculable pain, suffering, and heartache. Not only was my new husband habitually unfaithful and a flagrant liar, even more shockingly, it was suddenly revealed to me that he was also a criminal.

I have watched many TV documentaries and read many articles in magazines and newspapers about women who suddenly found out that their husband or partner was a criminal, and how they claimed to know nothing about it until suddenly all was revealed. There was part of me that always thought that they must have known, or they must have suspected something and seen some warning signs along the way. However, I now found myself in the same situation, and I was flabbergasted and taken completely by surprise by it all. I can honestly say that I had absolutely no idea about any of his criminal activity because he was so cunning in how he concealed things from me, and in what he chose to present to me. He even eventually admitted that he wanted me as his legitimate front to the world and community we lived in, the perfect cover story for his crimes. After living through several years of sheer hell and countless volatile arguments about his habitual infidelity, it was suddenly topped off like icing on a cake when he was arrested, which was how I found out about his criminal activity in one fell swoop.

It was surreal, it was like I was living a sleep paralysis nightmare straight out of one of the reality TV shows that cover this sort of thing. Not only was I suddenly alone again; my self-esteem had been battered beyond all recognition and I was at the lowest point I had ever been in my life. I had always thought of myself as being a strong and independent woman, but now I was emotionally flat on the floor and the walls of life seemed to be closing in on me from all sides.

My first divorce was amicable enough, and for broadly legitimate reasons as two people who still love each other simply grow apart when they do not share common goals. However, as a result of my husbands' criminal ways, in comparison, my second divorce was incredibly tumultuous, to say the least. The legal battles combined with criminal proceedings against him were an emotional roller coaster ride from hell as layer by layer his sociopathic criminal behaviour came painfully and embarrassingly to light.

Previously, despite his infidelity, I had never even considered ever leaving him, but now, with the turning of each metaphoric page, a new, darker, and even more sinister secret revealed the true nature of the man who I once loved. One moment, my life seemed to be full of all good things and set on a course for long-term happiness. The next moment, everything changed. Then in the blink of an eye, my sociopathic criminal husband had been deported back to his country of birth, and within the next few months, I also had to send my stepdaughter back to be with her mother in Gabon.

Suddenly, I was left in the empty house, with an empty life, and all I could do was try to pick up the pieces that were left. At that point, if I could have regained just a modicum of self-esteem it would have been a major achievement, but that was not going to happen at that time. Besides, it took all the effort I could muster to put on a brave face for the social world to gaze back upon as friends, neighbours, and even certain family members gossiped unkindly and knowingly about me. In addition, my two oldest biological children were now grown up and had flown the nest to follow their dreams and passions. So, for them at least, I had to somehow maintain the facade of being emotionally together and strong.

As you might imagine, this was not exactly a fun-filled time in my life. In addition, somehow, nagging away at me on the inside was the deepening hollow feeling that I had once again failed both my family and me at the same time. Emotionally, it was as if I were backed onto the ropes of a metaphoric boxing ring of life, just like Rocky Balboa was when

23

he was taking a battering from Clubber Lang or Ivan Drago in the fabulous movies. I also admit that at one point I even lost sight of hope. This is perhaps the lowest point that anyone can reach because the true darkness of the soul is not the absence of light, it is the absence of hope...

I have already admitted that by basic health standards when I entered into my second marriage, I was already a fatty. However, during and after my divorce and the legal battles, for over ten months my bodyweight ballooned beyond anything I had previously experienced. Interestingly, in retrospect, the surges in weight gain corresponded almost directly to match the depths of despair that I was feeling at any given time until very soon I weighed the heaviest I had ever been in my life.

Even more frighteningly, I even began to shift in my mind's eye to accept myself as being fat, and that my new size and shape was now normal for me. However, the only saving grace at the time was that I had changed jobs and was now working in the fashion industry, so I was always able to dress well and wear loose-fitting yet complimentary clothes that would cleverly hide the masses of excess weight I was now carrying. At first glance to the untrained eye, no one could tell just how fat and unfit I was.

The problem was that I knew, and it hurt me deeply to compound the emotional wounds I was still carrying from my divorce. In truth, I knew that I was now obese at well over 50 lbs heavier than my current weight as I write these words. Also, no matter how I dressed it up to accept myself and my body the way that I was, I was not truly happy and I certainly was not healthy. Soon, I even began having a tough time simply climbing stairs, walking only reasonable distances around shopping malls. I completely lacked both energy and enthusiasm, which then meant that I just wanted to sleep all the time. In short, I was a mess and I knew that this was a course that was set to end only one way, with diabetes, heart and circulatory disease, joint problems, and an ever-worsening sense of depression and an overall lack of self-esteem.

The Realisation that Being Fat But Fit is a Myth

This was the point in my life where I began to ask some important health questions and eventually perform research. This led me to conclude that when people say that they can be fat, but fit, it is a myth. I had heard the phrase, "They're fat but fit" on many occasions, and at face value, at the time it seemed plausible enough if someone was overweight and yet still regularly participated in some sort of sport, or outdoor physical activity of some kind.

However, today, after many more hours of research combined with looking beyond the boundaries of Minnesota and the USA in general, my earlier conclusions about this being a myth are now being validated by scientists, GPs, and clinicians all over the world.

The fat but fit theory suggests that carrying extra weight is not harmful if other metabolic factors are normal, this includes blood pressure and sugar levels. However, Professor Matthias Schulze, of the German Institute of Human Nutrition Potsdam-Rehbruecke, Nuthetal is just one of many leading scientists who have now exposed this theory as a myth with clinical evidence to support the claim.

Research that was carried out over 30 years, with over 90,000 women between 1980 and 2010, with updates from individuals participating every two years about their BMI (Base Metabolic Rate), their general metabolic health, medical histories, combined with data about their physical activity, exercise and lifestyle habits, ethnicity, family health histories, dietary choices, alcohol consumption, and smoking habits, because all of these factors may have influenced the research. The results found that even women who maintained what is commonly called metabolically healthy obesity for at least 20 years had a 57% higher than average risk of developing cardiovascular disease when compared with metabolically healthy women with a normal BMI and weight.

Interestingly, in comparison, women who were normal weight and yet fell into the metabolically unhealthy category were 2.5 times more likely to develop cardiovascular disease when compared to women with no metabolic abnormalities, and with a normal BMI and weight. However, the women who fell into the category of obesity yet considered metabolically healthy were still at substantially higher risk of developing cardiovascular disease by as much as a staggering 39%.

In addition, being overweight and particularly those who are obese are at a far higher risk of developing no less than twelve different types of cancers, including breast cancer. Interestingly, even as recently as March 2021, a report was released about a research study of 300,000 people undertaken by a team at Glasgow University. Unsurprisingly, the conclusion was simple; the fatter you are, the greater your risk of heart disease, cancer, type 2 diabetes, and strokes.

How is BMI (Body Mass Index) calculated? There are two formulas to calculate BMI and these depend upon if you use metric or imperial measurements. In metric, BMI = Weight (kg) / Height (m)^2 and in imperial, BMI = [Weight (lbs) / Height (inches)^2] x 703. To make It easier, the British NHS has a helpful calculator that can be found online at https://www.nhs.uk/live-well/healthy-weight/bmi-calculator/

The medically accepted BMI and weight categories are as follows.
- Underweight = BMI less than 18.5.
- Normal healthy weight = BMI between 18.5 and 24.9.
- Overweight = BMI between 25.0 and 29.9.
- Obese = BMI between 30.0 and 39.9.
- Morbidly obese = BMI 40.0 and above.

Dying to be Politically Correct

It is a sad fact that many people are now dying because of political correctness. This is because of how the messages conveyed by all media outlets encourage people, especially women, to be happy and satisfied with their bodies no matter how fat they are.

In fact, it is now almost taboo to even vaguely suggest that someone is overweight or needs to get fit because it may prove damaging to their feelings and mental health. This is of course, from the perspective of the perennially offended politically correct champions. At the same time, doctors, health professionals, and the government is also trying to get across the vitally important message about how there is an obesity epidemic, a diabetes epidemic, and a heart disease epidemic. This is because the subject must be discussed and addressed since so many people are now becoming seriously ill as a result.

Since we are now in this ridiculous position, what is the answer? How can anyone hope to solve such a serious, growing, and lethal problem simply because in the eyes of the emotionally weak it cannot be discussed?

This then begs two critically important questions. Is political correctness worth dying for? Is political correctness worth being ill for? The answer is NO to both, as far as I am concerned and hopefully for everyone with even a modicum of common sense. Any psychological damage that is done to those who are dithering, weak, and fragile just because they are told to lose weight and get fit is always going to be less harmful than the often-irreversible physical ravages of obesity, diabetes, cancers, and heart disease. The psychological impact of stating the obvious about the effects of obesity is also much less damaging than being dead as a result of the illnesses and diseases.

To put political correctness before good health to the point whereby people are needlessly developing serious diseases and illnesses is nothing more than totally and utterly stupid. However, some people seem to prefer being stupid, almost as if they possessed a stupidity gene. As always, things like this will be a personal choice. However, the biggest problem the terminally politically correct people have is that the science, biology, and physical mechanisms and side effects of obesity do not bow down and capitulate to political correctness.

If you are one of these people and you go against a plethora of scientific data and basic common sense about your health, then you only have yourself to blame when the inevitable happens and your body

27

begins to malfunction irreparably. This scenario is probably either in whole, or at least part, the Semmelweis Reflex in action. The Semmelweis Effect is a metaphor for the reflex-like tendency to reject new evidence or new knowledge simply because it contradicts the established, comfortable-feeling norms, beliefs, and/or paradigms. The term derives from the name of a Hungarian physician, Ignaz Semmelweis. Today, many supposedly intelligent people apparently seem to suffer from the Semmelweis Reflex. This means that some will never progress as fast or as far as they could if the politically correct types were more open-minded and able to process and embrace empirical data entirely without prejudice.

The Next Phase of My Life

At this point in my life, I had reached a stage where I was clinically obese, I felt awful, I was depressed, I was divorced again, and I knew that if I did not find some way to change my incredibly unhealthy lifestyle it would eventually kill me. By this time, and for completely different reasons to my own, my identical twin sister, Rhonda, had also gained weight to the point where she had become over 50 lbs over her optimal weight. Naturally, since we were identical twins, she is also the same height as me so being 50 lbs overweight did not look good. Thankfully, she was not emotionally bereft or battered as a result of a tumultuous divorce. Instead, her problems stemmed from years of overeating, excess drinking, and making generally poor lifestyle choices. So, she made a rational, positive life-changing decision. This was that she would lose weight and get fit. However, she did not simply mean 'fit' in terms of how average people perceive it, she had her sights set on achieving much more than that. She hired a coach and announced to the family that she would be entering a bodybuilding competition in the Figure Class within a year.

Once I had gotten over the initial surprise of my sister's declaration, I was extremely proud of her for wanting to lose her excess weight and build some muscle. However, I also hate to admit that I was completely sceptical about her ever achieving her target weight and competing on stage in a bikini in less than 12 months. Thankfully, I was proved wrong, because, after about 10 months of training several times each week with weights and following a strict diet, she had achieved her goals. She looked incredible, and I could hardly believe how much she had achieved.

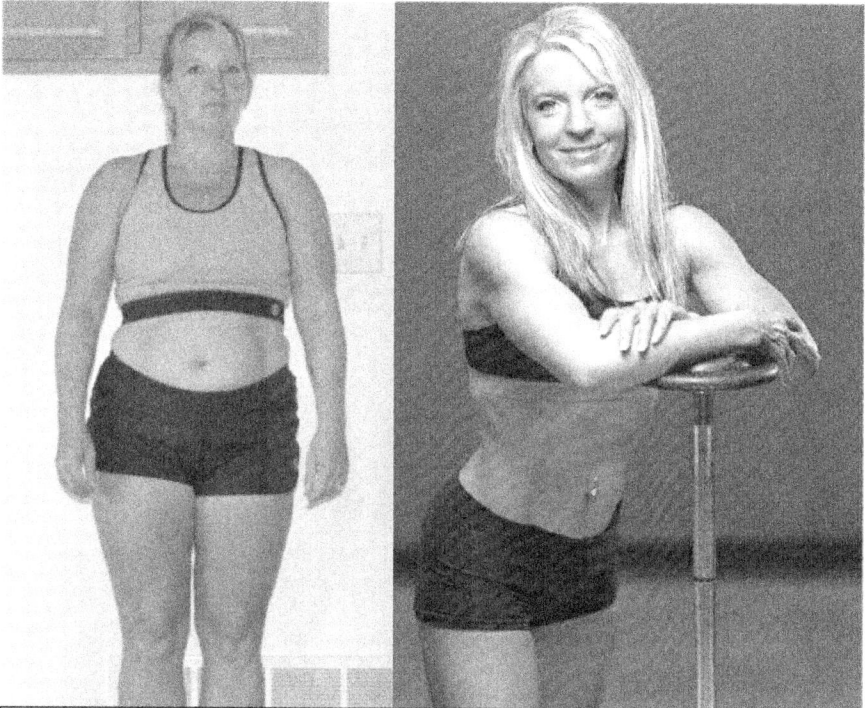

My twin sister, Rhonda, before she started (left) and (right) after just 10 months of training regularly and eating healthily.

This was when I had an epiphany moment because Rhonda's success made me realise that anybody can change the size, shape, and composition of their body to get into great shape IF they genuinely wanted to. Admittedly, I also knew that to do this would require willpower, determination, and some hard work, but I now knew that this was achievable if I genuinely wanted to succeed. I openly admit that my twin sister, Rhonda was my transformation inspiration, and I am eternally grateful to her for teaching me this important life lesson.

Becoming a Bikini Fitness Athlete

By this time, I knew two important things. One was that I was currently set on a course to face some serious and eventually life-threatening health issues combined with an abysmal level of fitness and emotional misery along the way. The other was that if I changed nothing in my life, then nothing would change. So, even though it took all the courage I could muster, I made a dramatic declaration. I committed to all my friends and family, together with my entire social media base, that I would not only lose all the excess weight that I gained, that I would get into peak physical shape and fitness, and that I would compete onstage in a major Bodybuilding Competition in the Bikini Fitness Class within 12 months. My declaration of intent must have been far more powerful than I realised because within a week one of my closest friends, Glenda Ama, decided to join me on my quest and compete in the same contest with me.

Next, came one of the toughest things I would face, this was to objectively assess every aspect of myself. I knew that if I stood any chance of succeeding then I could not afford to lie to myself about how fat, unfit, and out of shape I was, to begin with. If I had failed at this critical point, then I would have completely wasted my time and effort in the long term, and I would be merely pretending to get myself into shape. I cannot stress strongly enough just how important it is to objectively assess your starting point. A good analogy is that of a satellite navigation system. It can be the best system, the best hardware, the best software, the best of everything, BUT, if it cannot accurately pinpoint where you are at the start of your journey, then you will always fail to complete your journey. Lying to yourself about anything never works because you will always be the loser.

The objective self-assessment process was not in any way pleasant or easy, and since I had committed myself to a goal, I could not even lessen the emotional impact with a glass of wine! The fact was that if I were to not only compete but also stand a real chance of at least placing in the top five spots, then I would need to lose between 40 and 50 lbs of fat. Suddenly, instead of consuming what I objectively assessed to be between a typical 3 and 4 thousand calories a day, I had to reduce this to 1,200. To make this process easier, I decided to pre-cook all my meals for the coming week, and carefully weigh and portion everything out in advance in containers. This would then allow me to evenly spread out my food consumption every day so that I would be eating something roughly every 2 hours. This had the bonus of helping me to maintain a more constant level of blood sugar, combined with the sensation and satisfaction of eating food.

Next, I had to discipline myself to exercise regularly, and this meant setting time aside each day in my life schedule to go to the gym. It was obvious to me, even as a novice trainer, that this would mean that I had to make some significant adjustments to my lifestyle. I decided that the best time for me to get to the gym would be before work each day. Therefore, this meant me getting up at 0500 hrs every day and being at the gym, bright-eyes and bushy-tailed, no later than 0545 hrs because I had to be done and, on the road, to work by 0700 hrs, to deal with the 50-minute rush-hour commute to my office in Eden Prairie, MN. I am not a natural morning person, so before I had even started doing this, I already knew that this would be gruelling. I also knew that I would have to make sure that I was in bed and drifting off to sleep no later than 2130 hrs each evening if I wanted to ensure that I got enough quality sleep for rest and recovery. I also knew that the long-term benefits far outweighed any inconveniences and annoyances. It was a simple balance of choices that I knew I must make if I wanted to succeed in my quest. So, this became my new life. I must admit that when the alarm sounded at 0455 hrs on the first morning and I was getting up in the dark to exercise I felt a little like a female version of the character, Rocky Balboa.

Success in a thing like this rarely comes easily and without significant effort. This is why I have no time for people who belittle and dismiss the hard work, time, inconvenience, willpower and effort it took me to get into shape. And, yes, I had my fair share of encountering people like that along the way. Most people will be supportive along your fitness journey but don't be surprised that a few will be jealous. I had several people say to me, "When will go back to eating normally?" or "You don't need to lose any more weight, you like fine the way you are." To be honest, this actually motivated me even more.

According to ancient Chinese martial arts philosophy, the longest journey always starts with a single footstep that is the hardest to make. This is exactly how it was for me as I began my transformation journey because the first footstep was not easy on the first morning when the alarm sounded nauseatingly early. However, as each day passed, mercifully, it became progressively easier. So, I urge anyone facing a similar journey and commitment to have the courage to take that first step, no matter how challenging it might seem at the time.

The days soon turned into weeks, and the weeks soon turned into months, and since I had committed myself to the challenge, I never faltered or missed an exercise session or allowed my diet to slip. By this time, the cold, dark Minnesota winter had long since turned into spring, and then into early summer, and contest time for the Med City Muscle Classic taking place in Rochester, Minnesota! After only eight months I had done it! I had achieved all the goals I had set myself, and I confidently entered the contest in three categories, and amazingly, I earned 2nd, 3rd, and 4th place positions respectively in each class. I was elated, because only eight months before I was a blubbery, fat, podgy, obese mess of a woman who did not even look forward to seeing myself undressing to my underwear each evening to get ready for bed, let alone parade around confidently on stage in a skimpy bikini in a bodybuilding contest.

It was about one month before this contest that I met the man who is now my husband. We first made a connection because he was a coach in exercise, strength and conditioning who had once helped to train the 4-time World's Strongest Man, Jon Pall Sigmarsson of Iceland, and a host of other champion sportspeople and martial artists. He was incredibly supportive and gave me some excellent training tips that made a huge difference to my overall progress.

After the contest was over, I had well and truly caught the 'stay in shape' bug. I also knew that it would always be much easier to maintain sight of my contest-ready body shape rather than let it all slip away again by reverting to making poor lifestyle choices again. Therefore, I committed to enter another contest the following year, the Milwaukee Muscle Madness event in Wisconsin. It was around this time when my new man had become my fiancee, and when he began explaining how I could make even greater progress in terms of muscle size and shape by doing something I thought at the time seemed to be counterintuitive.

The Appliance of Science Prevented Me from Confusing Activity with Accomplishment

In short, Brian explained that less could result in more. What he was referring to was the length of time I was spending exercising in a gym could be too much, especially since by this time I was in my mid-40s, and heading north of that, to my 50s. He explained that exercise is a stimulus intended to trigger a physical response, namely maintaining or building muscle, maintaining muscle tone, and maintaining an elevated BMR, or Base Metabolic Rate. You need just enough stimulation to trigger all the desirable physical processes, and not too much so that it triggers some less desirable processes. This also meant that there must be sufficient rest time so that our bodies and recover positively. It can be remarkably easy to overtrain, especially as we get older, and if we do, then this can stress the body and instead of generating a positive physical response, it can trigger a negative one.

It is well researched and known that people who exercise for prolonged periods and extreme endurance athletes who create high levels of physiological stress, are collectively at a greater risk of suffering temporary immunodepression and have a higher risk of contracting an infection. More importantly, this type of exercise makes people much more susceptible to contracting upper respiratory tract infections due to overtraining while their immune systems are depressed. In addition, the stress hormone, cortisol. Cortisol is a naturally occurring hormone, secreted by the adrenal glands, that plays a key part in how the body responds to stress. Cortisol is involved in the regulation of the following functions, and several others:

- △ Inflammatory response.
- △ Immune function.
- △ Blood pressure.
- △ Glucose metabolism.
- △ Insulin release.

Cortisol is released by the adrenal glands in response to stress, or fear as part of our natural fight or flight response. If we are suddenly faced with a threat our body responds to prepare us to meet the challenges of that perceived threat. In the brain, the amygdala signals the hypothalamus, which in turn triggers other mechanisms, including the release of hormones including adrenaline and cortisol. However, too much cortisol can be bad for you in several ways. If our cortisol levels remain too high for too long due to stress, then it can trigger many adverse effects, including the following.

- △ Decreased muscle tissue.
- △ Increased abdominal fat.
- △ Decreased bone density.
- △ Decreased immune and inflammatory responses.
- △ Suppressed thyroid function.
- △ Increased blood pressure.
- △ Increased levels of LDL, or bad cholesterol.
- △ Decreased levels of HDL, or good cholesterol.
- △ Blood sugar imbalances, including hyperglycemia.

In short, increased levels of cortisol in the blood will work directly against every aspect of what you are trying too hard to achieve, a little like trying to sail a ship directly into the wind. Therefore, if one does not achieve the correct balance of exercise as a stimulus in terms of how long, hard, and intensely it is performed, then it can easily result in the body becoming stressed and producing too much cortisol. This is because anthropologically the body cannot recognise the difference between being chased by a sabre-toothed tiger and the stress caused by too much exercise. As we age, our stress tolerance trigger level reduces. This means that to ensure we are not confusing activity with accomplishment by training in such a way that it causes our body to work against us, we must temper what we do accordingly.

It does not matter what exercise you used to do years ago, or how long you could do it for back then, regrettably, it is a simple truth that the older you get the less you can do at all levels. To maintain optimal progress, what you do and how you do it becomes more important than ever. Ideally, instead of exercising for extended periods, workout sessions should become brief, intense, and focused. All of this becomes even more important as women approach, and then try to navigate their way through menopause. They can emerge from it while still maintaining as much of their youthful, vigorous, and sexy appearance as possible. The whole approach to exercise, weight, shape, Body Mass Index and muscle tone etc. becomes more about managing it all within the ever-shifting parameters of ageing.

Brian suggested that I should dramatically reduce the long exercise sessions I had been performing leading up to my first contest, and start training smarter. He suggested that I should employ his TRISOmetric™ exercise system instead. The TRISOmetric™ exercise system is a combination of three scientifically proven techniques into a single unified approach. The three techniques are, 1) Isometric exercise 2) Minimum triple point isometric exercise along the ROM, or Range Of Motion of each limb, and 3) Super-slow calisthenic exercise to follow the isometric portion. The system also incorporates other scientifically proven aspects including a specific length of time taken between each exercise, and Ultra Short Ultra High-intensity bursts of exercise etc.

Since isometric exercise is one of the most efficient and result-producing in terms of the ratio of the effort expended and results gained. Therefore, when multiple isometric exercise points were employed in the same exercise and then combined with super-slow callisthenics, it made complete sense to me. It all worked amazingly well. Previously, for my first contest, I had trained the traditional way and spent at least an hour in the gym every day with only one day off each week. Since the TRISOmetric™ exercise system can be made so challenging, it did not mean that I had to use weights and exercise in a gym for every workout. It was very easy to use a portable total-body gym device such as a pair of Iso-Bows® that enabled me to have a workout virtually anywhere. Since I was no longer bound and restricted by the requirement for me to always be near a well-equipped gym each day, I was not only able to exercise anywhere I chose, I also regained the unfettered freedom to travel I had not experienced in well over a year!

In addition, in preparing for my first contest, I had consumed an average of 150 grams of protein each day, which had embarrassingly adverse side effects on my digestive system. Now, for my second contest, I was training at home most of the time, my workout sessions lasted no longer than an average of twenty minutes every other day, and since I was consuming about 70 grams of protein per day on average, I was suffering no embarrassing adverse side effects from my diet. The only side effect I can report was a positive one, which was that I found controlling my weight, Body Mass Index, and overall fat levels far easier than before doing things the traditional way.

The result of all these dramatic changes in my approach to diet and exercise was that I placed first in my class in the Minnesota Muscle Mayhem contest held in Duluth in 2016. After finally believing I had mastered the perfect workout program, menopause hit me like a ton of bricks. After 4 years of consistent workouts and maintaining my weight, once I hit 50, my workouts were no longer working. My weight was slowly creeping back up. I soon found out that I was over-exercising! My 30-minute workouts were just too much, even though I enjoyed them immensely. I needed to dial right back and I started researching and found that it was important to maintain muscle but also, not workout too much to increase my cortisol. Not only that, I had to cut back my calorie intake even more.

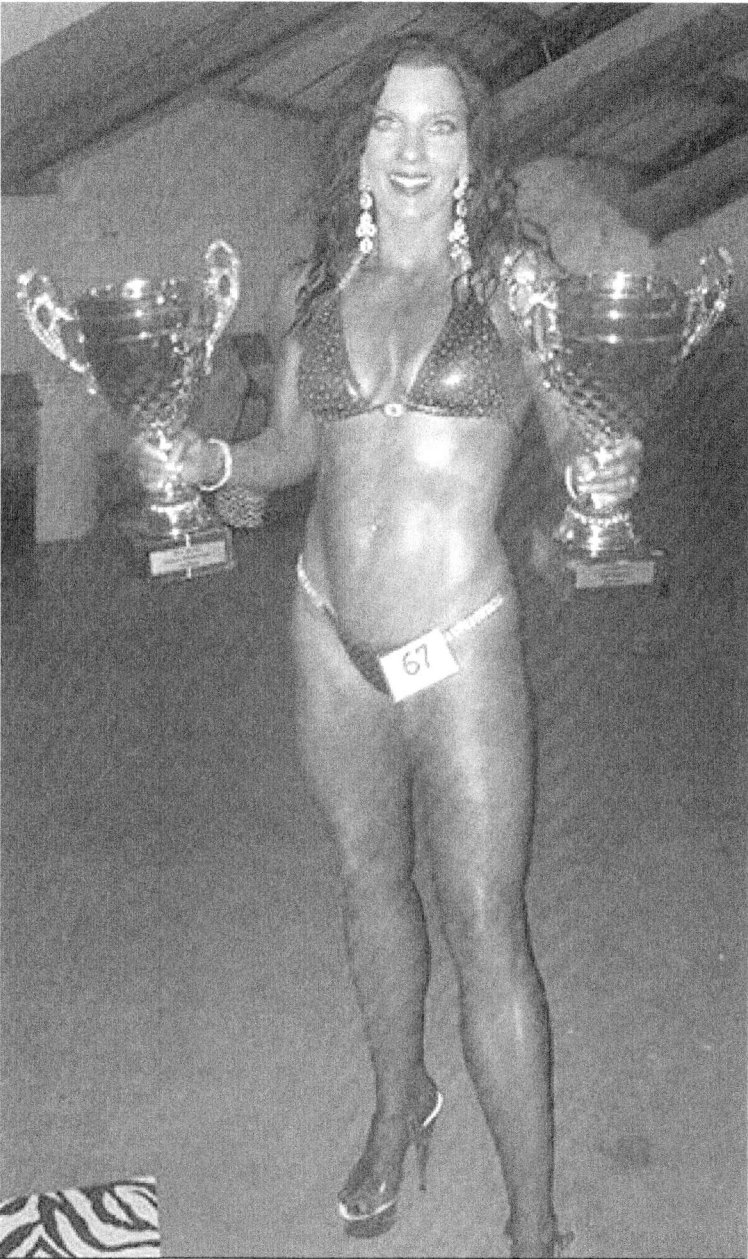

This is me, a multi-trophy winner, after performing a structured TRISOmetric exercise plan, and at times, as little as 70-Seconds of Exercise a Day.

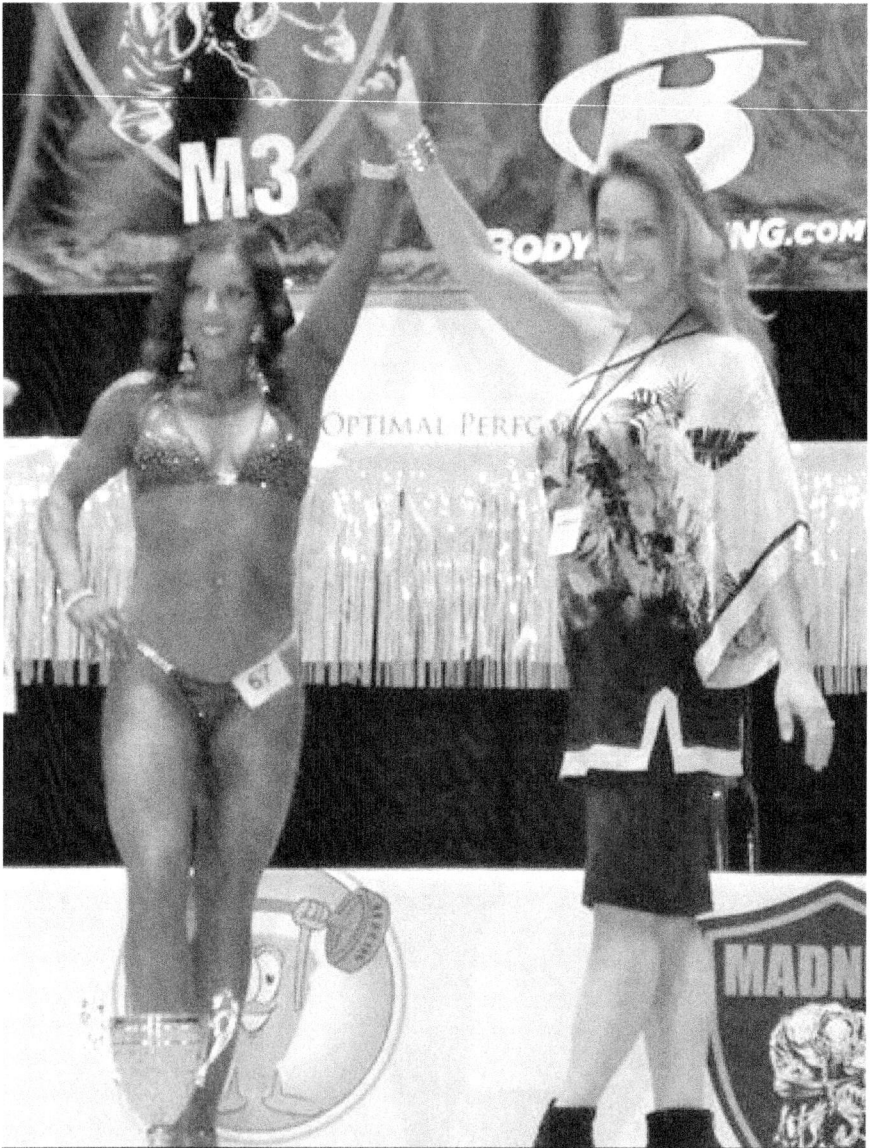

On stage when I was winning multiple trophies.

The Great Protein Myth

At this point, I feel that I should elaborate more on why Brian suggested that I change my overall type of diet and the previous approach to how much protein I should consume. When I first started training I hired a coach to devise both an exercise routine and nutrition plan. In hindsight, unsurprisingly since he had been trained traditionally, he recommended that I consume as much protein as possible. Who was I to argue with him? After all, he should know – right? It seems that the traditional approach to calculating an athlete's daily protein requirements was seriously flawed.

Brian explained it thoroughly, and since I knew that his writing on the subject had been praised by a mutual and well-respected friend, Dr Joseph M. Gryskiewicz, a Clinical Professor at the University of Minnesota Academic Health Center and a Fellow of the American College of Surgeons. I remember the conversation clearly and how he agreed with Brian, his calculations, approach, and his choice of protein source which was vegan. It seems that the obsession amongst bodybuilders and those who exercise in general to consume ever-increasing quantities of protein is typically fuelled by the myriad of confusing magazine articles, poorly trained coaches, and advertisements that all promote the supposed need to consume massive amounts of protein. Amazingly, despite a mass of empirical data suggesting against it, The Academy of Nutrition and Dietetics reports that bodybuilders require about 0.63 to 0.77 grams of protein per pound of body weight each day and that 1.4 to 1.8 grams of protein per kilogram are required to build muscle mass.

It is just a fact that human muscle is composed of between 16% and 25% protein, depending upon the research study type of the sample used. However, most research averaged between 20% and 22%, with the rest of the muscle being composed of around 70% water, carbohydrates, and fat. If the body tissue you are seeking to build is not composed of anything more than about 22% protein, then it is just stupid to stuff yourself with massive quantities of protein, in the pathetic and misguided belief that more is always better. More importantly, consuming too much protein will slow down your body shaping and bodybuilding progress. This is because your body will be desperately trying to process the continued protein overdose it is being force-fed.

Also, research indicates that the average human male under optimal training conditions, and without the use of drugs, can only usually gain about 10 lbs of lean muscle per year. Naturally, a female would gain somewhat less. Since one pound of muscle contains 600 calories, then 10 lbs of muscle mass equate to a value of 6000 calories. Therefore, logic and science indicate that only an additional 6000 calories should be consumed to build all the lean muscle mass that a human can gain each year. Naturally, the additional 6000 calories should be consumed gradually throughout the year. That is an average of only 16.44 extra calories per day. More importantly, only four of those calories needs to be from a protein source because muscle is approximately only 20-22% protein by composition. Surprise, surprise! Mother Nature's natural foods already had the correct nutritional balance right after all.

In addition to this, the famous, and eminent sports scientist, Dr Ellington Darden, gathered research data that supported this concept. Since that time, he has pointed out on many occasions that it is water and carbohydrates that are the most important components of building muscle, not protein. Again, this is simply because of applying logic about water and carbohydrates being the bulk of what human muscle tissue is composed of. Dr Ellington Darden's advice to some of the greatest and most successful bodybuilders of all time was to consume a diet of between 60-70% carbohydrates, 15-25% fats, and 15-25% protein. Therefore, he advised that a 200 lb bodybuilder should consume about 0.36 grams of protein per lb of body weight, in other words about 72 grams.

Current research indicates that the optimum amount of protein the average human should consume with each meal should be an absolute maximum of around 30 grams. It also indicates that an average person who does not exercise should consume about 46 grams of protein per day for women and 56 grams per day for men. Despite all of our research, we have still not been able to find a study showing that even consuming only the recommended minimum RDA of 10% protein, which is 10% of your overall daily calorie intake, has any adverse effects on an athlete's muscle growth or sports performance. Therefore, consuming plant-based protein within the so-called recommended mid-range, which is between 10% and 25% protein of your overall daily calorie intake, is still more than enough to build muscle even for a high-performance athlete. However, our recommendation would be to consume a maximum of about 22% protein, entirely from plant-based sources, and with a complete amino acid complex.

Menopause – My Next Frontier

With a first-place contest win under my belt, I felt elated, and even though I say so myself, I looked amazing. However, by this time, I was fast approaching the big 5-0, and, since my twin sister had already shown the first signs, I knew that menopause was not far away. This is not an easy thing to face for any woman because for many, it is inseparably interwoven with who we are as women both biologically and emotionally. This meant that my journey through menopause could well be a personal challenge that, in its own way, could be every bit as great as any challenge that I had faced in my life to date. I also knew that even physically and emotionally life would be a journey that ran a little like a waveform along a timeline, one of peaks and troughs.

Since it would probably be virtually impossible to eliminate it completely, then the best strategy would be to minimise the waveform. This would make the peaks (if there were that many) not quite so high, and the troughs not quite so low. Even though I already knew quite a bit about menopause, I also knew that the sources of my information were primarily from my mother and other women I knew who were either going through it or had already gone through it. Since none of them was a medical doctor or scientist, it meant that I must now turn the focus of my attention onto researching all about the looming 'enemy' from reputable scientific sources. Hearsay, rumour, and talk of grandmas remedies were no good for me unless they were backed by proven science. To begin my new voyage of exploration, I dialled it right back to the beginning. I wanted to identify scientifically, exactly what menopause is, what might or might not happen, why certain things happen, when I should expect things to happen, and the biological mechanics of everything involved.

The term menopause technically refers to a point in time that follows one year after the last menstruation occurs. Menopause is the polar opposite of menarche, which is the time when a girl will have her first period. The word, menopause literally means the "end of monthly cycles, periods or menstruation" and comes from the Greek word "pausis" meaning "pause" and "mēn" meaning "month". The word "menopause" was specifically coined for human females where the end of fertility is indicated by the permanent cessation of monthly menstruation.

Physiologically, menopause happens because of a decrease in the ovaries' production of the hormones estrogen and progesterone. There have been rare cases reported when a woman's ovaries stop working at a comparatively very early age. Somewhat alarmingly, this premature ovarian failure can be anywhere between the age of puberty and age 40 and affects up to 2% of women.

The transition into menopause, or perimenopause, typically lasts for 7 years, however, it can sometimes be as long as 14 years. Other research has indicated that this transition phase can be anything between 4 years and 10, so this is not fixed. The term perimenopause "around the menopause", and refers to the menopause transition years before the date of the final period.

To confuse matters slightly, premenopause (note the slight spelling change from using the letter 'i' to the letter 'e' in the word) means the years leading up to the last period and starts before the monthly cycles become noticeably irregular. This is when the levels of reproductive hormones are becoming more varied as they decrease and the effects of hormone withdrawal are present.

Symptoms of
Menopause

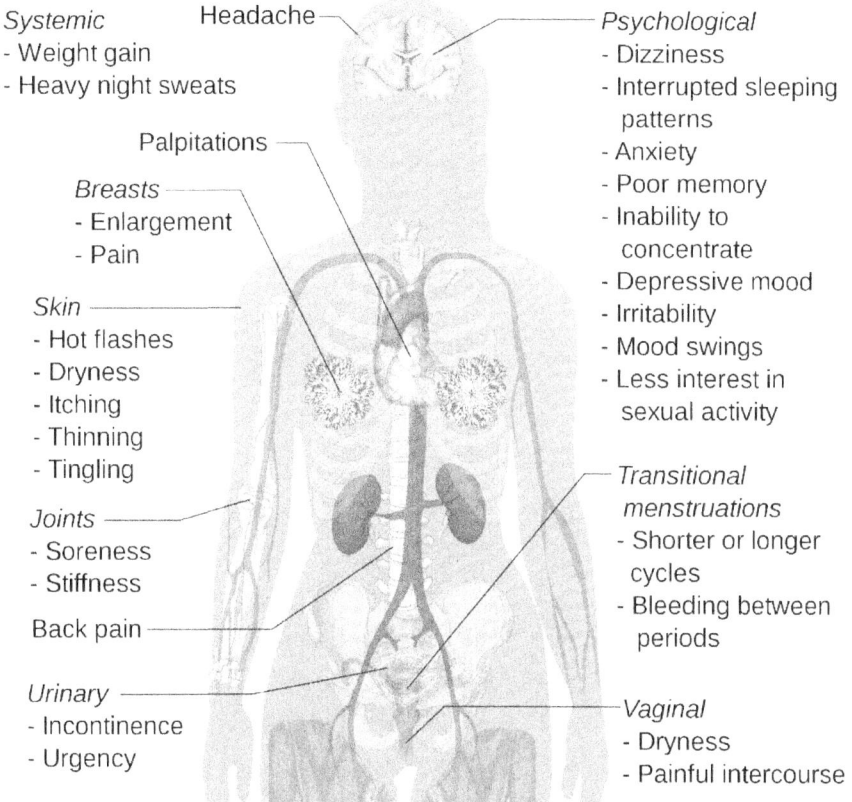

Systemic
- Weight gain
- Heavy night sweats

Headache

Palpitations

Breasts
- Enlargement
- Pain

Skin
- Hot flashes
- Dryness
- Itching
- Thinning
- Tingling

Joints
- Soreness
- Stiffness

Back pain

Urinary
- Incontinence
- Urgency

Psychological
- Dizziness
- Interrupted sleeping
  patterns
- Anxiety
- Poor memory
- Inability to
  concentrate
- Depressive mood
- Irritability
- Mood swings
- Less interest in
  sexual activity

*Transitional
menstruations*
- Shorter or longer
  cycles
- Bleeding between
  periods

Vaginal
- Dryness
- Painful intercourse

Symptoms of Menopause - Picture Credit Mikael Häggström

However, most research suggests that menopause typically occurs between 49 and 52 years of age, depending upon several factors that include genetics, lifestyle, and diet. Roughly 50% of women report having their last period between the ages of 47 and 55, with approximately 80% having their last period between 44 and 58 years of age. The average age of women to have their the last period is as follows.

- ⚠ The United Kingdom 52 years.
- ⚠ The United States 51 years.
- ⚠ Australia 51 years.

△ Ireland 50 years.
△ India and the Philippines 44 years.

Menopause is the time in a woman's life when her menstrual periods stop permanently so she is no longer able to have children. Also, doctors frequently diagnose menopause as having occurred if a woman has not had any menstrual bleeding for a year. For some women, pre-menopausal problems such as experiencing painful periods and/or endometriosis can significantly improve after going through menopause and emerging on the other side.

In addition, menopause is typically accompanied by a decrease in hormone production by the ovaries, adipose tissues, and placenta. In particular, there is a decline in estrogen or oestrogen levels that is a sex hormone responsible for the development and regulation of the female reproductive system and secondary sex characteristics.

Technically, for women who have had surgery to remove their uterus but still have their ovaries, menopause may be considered to have occurred when they had the surgery. If a woman has her uterus removed, then menopause symptoms usually begin much earlier than if her uterus had been left in place, at an average of 45 years of age. However, the removal of the uterus is typically for medical reasons of such importance that they outweigh it preventing a woman from being able to have children and making menopause occur.

Early in the menopause process the cycles usually remain regular. However, in the years leading up to the onset of menopause women typically experience a certain degree of somewhat irregular periods. A period may occasionally be missed, others might be longer in duration, or shorter, some might be heavier and others lighter in terms of blood flow. As the menopause process progresses, it is the interval between cycles that changes as it begins to lengthen and ovulation may not occur with each cycle

Around this time when the first tell-tale symptoms begin to show, most women begin to experience hot flushes, or flashes, depending upon the type of transatlantic vernacular being used. The length of time a hot flush lasts varies but is typically between as little as 30 seconds to as long as ten to 15 minutes. In addition, hot flushes are usually associated with other symptoms including profuse sweating to the point whereby a woman feels that the heating in a room has been turned up full blast. Other common symptoms include shivering due to the intense feeling of coldness, and the reddening and irritation of the skin. The latter can sometimes make a woman feel as though not only her cheeks are flushed, but her entire face has suddenly become bright red as a result.

Oddly, a hot flush often seems to be triggered by an external influence causing an imbalance. This could be something as mundane as taking a sip of wine that previously would have had no effect, but during menopause it annoyingly does.

The effect of hot flushes can be minimised by taking a few simple steps that include avoiding caffeine and alcohol, stopping smoking, and wherever possible, sleeping in a cooler than usual room. I found that using lighter cotton bed sheets and a simple strategically directed fan running overnight helped me enormously.

Thankfully, the hot flushes usually stop within 12 to 24 months of their onset. However, in truth, the hot flushes sometimes feel like they will never end, and experiencing only a few months of them can feel like an eternity. As if all this were not enough, other extremely annoying symptoms include the following.

- Poor, troubled, and interrupted sleep patterns.
- Heavy night sweats.
- Wide-ranging mood swings.
- The inability to concentrate.
- Depressed mood.
- Often extreme irritability.
- Poor memory.
- Headaches.
- Anxiety.

△ Embarrassing vaginal dryness.
△ Lack of energy.
△ Heart palpitations.
△ Breast enlargement and/or pain.
△ Urinary incontinence and/or urgency.
△ Weight gain.
△ Joint soreness.
△ General stiffness and also back pain.
△ Tingling skin.
△ Itchy skin.
△ Reduced interest in sexual activity.

Certain external influences often cause menopause to occur earlier in a woman's life, these include smoking tobacco which can cause menopause to begin 1 to 3 years earlier than average, certain types of chemotherapy, radiotherapy, oophorectomy, hysterectomy, and having surgery to remove both ovaries. Since coeliac disease can be present without the common gastrointestinal symptoms, timely recognition and go undiagnosed, leading to a risk of long-term complications. Coeliac disease that is either untreated or has not been diagnosed can cause menopause to start earlier than average. However, early diagnosis and treatment of the disease typically afford women a more normal duration of their fertility.

An official medical diagnosis of menopause having begun is typically not normally sought, or indeed needed for obvious reasons. However, it can be medically detected and confirmed by measuring hormone levels in either the blood or urine. Similarly, specific treatment for menopause is also not needed. If a woman is experiencing certain serious issues relating to menopause, then some symptoms can be alleviated and improved with certain treatments.

The most commonly prescribed medications that have been found to help include MHT or Menopausal Hormone Therapy. However, since there are now concerns about side effects, even though MHT was once commonly prescribed it is now only recommended for women experiencing significant symptoms. Other medications that can help include gabapentin, selective serotonin reuptake inhibitors, and clonidine. There is tentative evidence suggesting that phytoestrogens such as those found in soya beans and related products can help.

Unsurprisingly, to some degree, menopause always has a psychological effect on women. The degree of this effect varies, and to some may even be almost imperceptible, but there is always an effect. For some, there is a huge sense of happiness and relief because they no longer have to worry about having periods or using birth control. For other women, there is a huge sense of loss about them losing their fertility and subsequently how they identify themselves as a woman. For other women. In fact, menopause can lead to many women becoming significantly clinically depressed as a result.

Pre-menopause, these women may have never experienced a depressing moment, but when menopause hits it can be like a head-on emotional express train collision. A high percentage of women report that during the menopause years they experience what they describe as having their lowest emotional sense of well-being in their lives. Again, unsurprisingly, the many hormonal level fluctuations throughout the body facilitate chemical changes to the neurotransmitters in the brain are linked to depressed senses of well-being because they trigger wide-ranging mood changes and subsequent emotional roller-coaster rides that accompany them.

It is widespread for women to report greatly decreased libido around, during and after menopause. In addition, some report feeling deeply depressed and saddened because they are no longer fertile, and getting pregnant is then impossible. In respect of children, the timeline of life brings with it significant markers such as having children leave the family home to live alone, attend a college or university and make their own way in the world. This can cause what is known as Empty Nest Syndrome and is a feeling of varying degrees of grief and loneliness parents experience due to feeling a loss of purpose and the subsequent adjustments they make in their lives as a result. This syndrome is especially common in full-time mothers. Next comes a sense of finality of loss when the children get married, this is then enhanced by the birth of grandchildren. These things, either consciously or subconsciously, psychologically label people as being middle-aged. Also, when great-grandchildren are born, people similarly shift to transition into old age. Each of these transition phases brings with it certain senses and feelings of ever-increasing loss, long-term hopelessness, and depression.

Interestingly, research indicates that a melatonin supplement in perimenopausal women can help offset many of these negative emotional states. This is because it improves gonadotropin levels and overall thyroid function. Gonadotropins are hormones secreted by the placenta in pregnant humans and are central to the endocrine system that regulates normal growth, sexual development. The overall effect of the supplementation can include the restoration of fertility and menstruation, while at the same time helping to prevent depression associated with menopause. More in-depth studies need to be performed into this supplementation and mechanism, but it appears to be very promising.

Regarding menopause, HRT or Hormone Replacement Therapy is when estrogen is used by women without a uterus, and when estrogen combined with progestin is used by women who have an intact uterus. HRT is perhaps the most commonly known treatment and is effective for menopausal symptoms such as hot flushes. HRT is commonly delivered as a skin patch, however, research has indicated that it appears to increase the risk of strokes and blood clots. Therefore, it is often recommended that is used for the shortest time and in the lowest effective dose possible. This also makes HRT frequently unsuitable for women who are at increased risk of cardiovascular disease, thromboembolic disease due to obesity or those with a history of venous thrombosis, or for those with increased risk of some types of cancer.

By adding testosterone to the HRT it has a positive effect on sexual function, especially in postmenopausal women. However, the downside of this can be side effects such as acne, annoying hair growth especially on the face and a reduction in HDL or High-Density Lipoprotein which is known as the good type of cholesterol.

Men and Menopause

Men are not immune to menopause, and since the word itself contains the word "men" many women argue that this is part of why it is so challenging for them to face. Joking aside, few men seem to realise that they go through a similar change that is commonly called by the media "the male menopause" and/or "andropause" and are labels that are unfortunately somewhat misleading. This is because both imply that men experience a sudden change in hormone levels similar to what women experience in menopause, which they do not because the transition for men is more gradual yet equally unavoidable.

The decrease in libido men experience is as a result of age is sometimes colloquially referred to as the "penopause" and is technically called LOH, or Late-Onset Hypogonadism, or TDS which is also referred to as Testosterone Deficiency Syndrome. LOH/TDS is a condition in older men that is the result of a gradual decrease in testosterone levels of about 1% per year. This is then characterized by the decreased desire for sex, fewer spontaneous erections, and even erectile dysfunction. However, this is another avenue of exploration, that is associated with, but not pertinent to my main exploration of women and menopause.

Osteoporosis and Menopause

Osteoporosis literally means "porous bone" and it is a systemic skeletal disorder characterized by low bone mass, physical strength, micro-architectural deterioration of bone tissue leading to bone fragility, and the consequent risk of an increase in fractures. Unfortunately, osteoporosis is a silent disease because it often begins and then progresses without any perceivable symptoms or pain. It typically remains unknown until the bones become so weak that a sudden fall, bump, fracture, or break occurs, usually in the back or hips, or most painfully when a vertebra collapses. If a vertebra collapses, this could easily manifest itself initially

49

as back pain, and osteoporosis might only be discovered upon medical examination. A collapsed vertebrae may also result in the loss of a person's normal height or spinal deformities such as stooped posture. Concerningly, the medical profession still does not know the exact cause of osteoporosis, however, they do know how the disease develops.

In simple terms, bones are living, growing tissue with an outer shell of dense bone encasing the inner sponge-like trabecular bone. When a bone is weakened by osteoporosis, the "holes" of the inner sponge-like trabecular bone grow larger and become more numerous, which in turn, weakens the internal structure. Until about age 30, people normally build more bone than they lose. As part of the ageing process, bone breakdown eventually begins to outpace bone build-up, which results in bone loss. When a certain point in the bone loss process is reached, a person has osteoporosis.

The next obvious question is, how is osteoporosis related to menopause? Unfortunately, there is a direct connection because of the decrease in oestrogen during perimenopause and menopause. In addition, early menopause, which is somewhere before the age of 45, and any prolonged periods during which hormone levels are low and menstrual periods are absent and/or infrequent can cause loss of bone mass.

Women who are at any stage of menopause, especially the mid, later and post stages and those over the age of 50, have the highest risk of developing osteoporosis. This is compounded because women, especially petite ones, naturally have comparatively thinner bones than men, which, in and of itself, compounds their increased risk of having osteoporosis. Studies show that when compared to men of similar age, women are 4 times more likely to develop osteoporosis. Men with small, thin bones are naturally at a higher risk.

In addition, your genetics are indicators of potential risk factors for osteoporosis. If you do not already know, it is worth checking to see if your parents or grandparents have had any signs of osteoporosis. They may not call it osteoporosis, so check for signs such as someone suffering a fractured hip after a comparatively minor fall. If there are any indicators in your family tree, then you may be at greater risk of developing the disease. Similarly, research has shown that Caucasian and Asian women are more likely to develop osteoporosis and twice as likely to develop hip fractures when compared to Afro-Caribbean women. Sadly, Afro-Caribbean women who suffer a serious fracture such as that of the hips in later years, have a higher mortality rate.

There are several painless and accurate tests that your doctor can perform to check your bone density health and for osteoporosis. These include BMD or Bone Mineral Density tests, low radiation X-rays, and simply keeping an accurate track of bone measurements over a period of time. All of these are worth considering because it is better to be forewarned so that you can take a proactive approach to the effects of ageing in general and osteoporosis in particular.

The commonly accepted medical treatments for osteoporosis include HRT or Hormone Replacement Therapy, as well as food supplements of calcium and vitamin D. In addition, weight-bearing resistance exercises are also effective in slowing and in some cases even stop the development of osteoporosis. Traditional medical advice will suggest that eating enough foods high in calcium throughout your life will help to build and maintain strong, healthy bones. We wholeheartedly agree with this.

However, the medical profession and even many nutritionists are traditional in their approach and have failed to embrace the more modern in-depth studies and comparisons. They will suggest that to get the circa 1,000 milligrams (mg) RDA or Recommended Daily Allowance that adults with an average risk of developing osteoporosis require or for postmenopausal women and those in the higher sick category, circa 1,200 milligrams (mg) per day, they should consume more milk and dairy products. Choosing any dairy product as a source of calcium is a terrible idea, and we shall explain why shortly. Hopefully, they will also recommend the consumption of lots of vegetable sources including the following:

- Dark green leafy vegetables such as broccoli, kale, and Brussels sprouts.
- Soybeans and related products.
- Beans.
- Peas.
- Lentils
- Nuts such as almond and Brazil.
- Certain seeds such as sesame.
- Grains such as amaranth and teff, that are gluten-free.
- Seaweed including wakame and kelp.
- Some fruit such as raw figs, oranges, blackberries, and raspberries.
- Calcium-fortified plant-based yoghurts.
- Blackstrap molasses.

Dairy as a Source of Calcium

Refreshingly even the Harvard School of Public health now suggests that people look away from the dairy aisle in supermarkets when they are searching for foods that are high in calcium. (see: https://www.hsph.harvard.edu/nutritionsource/what-should-you-eat/calcium-and-milk/)

The simple, and perhaps shocking fact is that dairy is a terrible source of calcium for humans. Where does a cow get the dietary calcium that it needs? It gets it from the plants that it eats, of course. Also, since many plants are an excellent source of magnesium, they allow the calcium contained in them to be easily digested, absorbed, and readily used by the body. The calcium contained in cow's milk is relatively useless because it does not have sufficient magnesium to allow it all to be fully absorbed and used by the human body. In fact, it only has enough magnesium content to allow approximately 11% of what is ingested to be properly absorbed.

It is also interesting to note the nations that produce and consume the largest amounts of dairy foods are also the nations where the population suffers from the highest levels of osteoporosis. Look at the data relating to this for Holland, the Scandinavian countries, New Zealand, the United States and Germany. The facts are plain to see, and they are easy to understand. It does not take Sherlock Holmes to connect the dots about this and form a logical link.

Also, in general, dairy products are rich in casein, the milk protein which is linked to causing cancer. This fact alone should be a good enough reason to avoid dairy foods. Milk also contains growth hormones. The most powerful human growth hormone is identical to the most powerful bovine growth hormone. That same hormone instructs every cell in the human body to grow. This is one reason why bodybuilders love dairy products so much, and especially whey protein.

However, the growth hormone instructs every cell in the human body to grow, including cancer cells. There have been many studies conducted about this, and they all conclude the direct link between consuming dairy products and cancer production in humans. Research by Dr T. Colin Campbell even showed that casein, which is 87% of the protein found in milk, promoted ALL the stages of the cancer process. The link between casein and cancer was so conclusive that in clinical tests, scientists could turn cancer production in rats on and off by simply altering the amount of casein in their diet. Research showed that a diet that comprised more than 5% of casein turned on cancer production, and diets that comprised less than 5%, down to zero casein, turned off cancer production.

Overall, consuming dairy products makes your whole body weaker and increasingly ill. There is also clear scientific evidence that despite what the dairy producers say, dairy products are related to diseases and illnesses such as diabetes, joint problems, allergies, heart disease, constipation, asthma, rheumatoid arthritis, lymphoma, and multiple sclerosis.

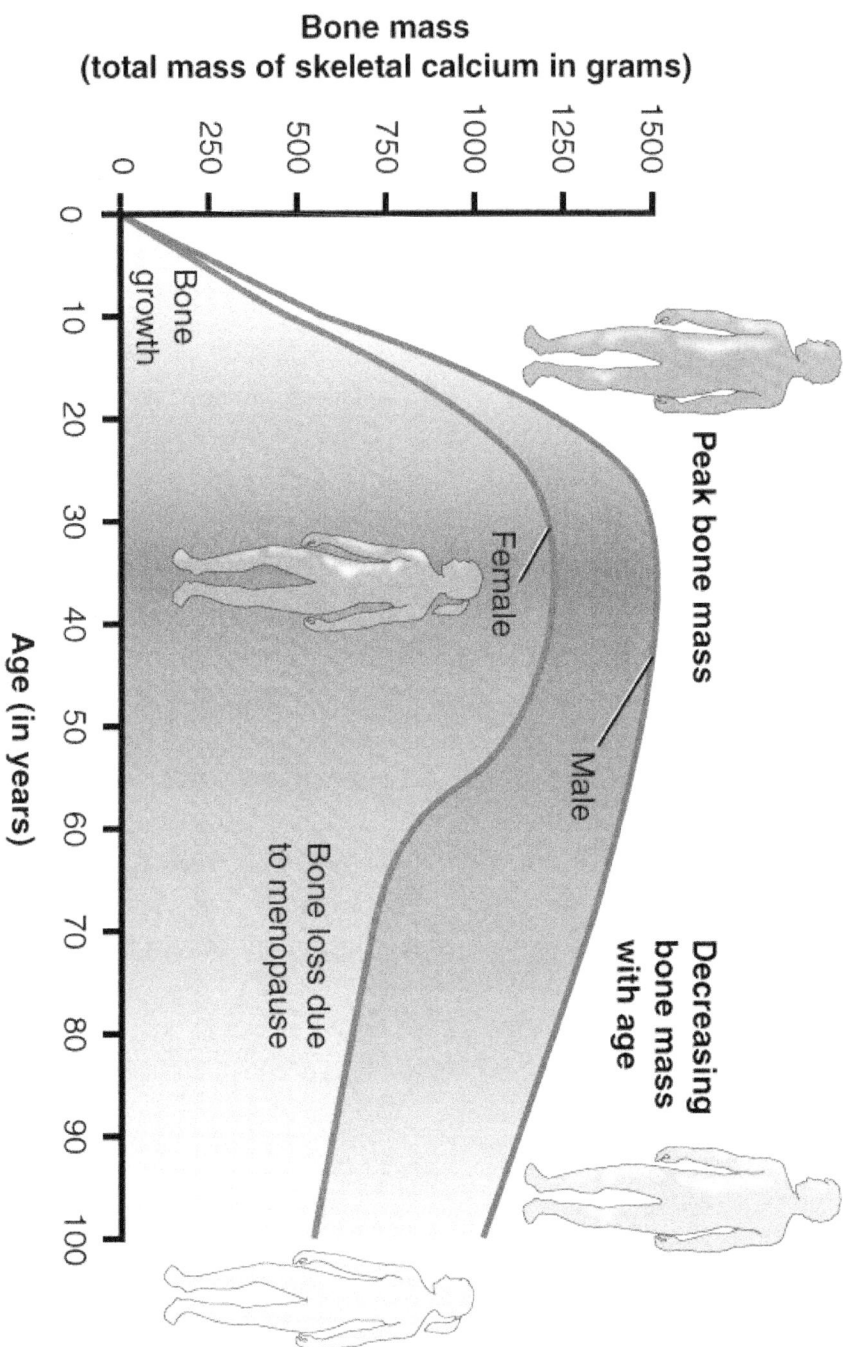

Age and Bone Mass - Picture Credit OpenStax College

Dairy and Osteoporosis

We now know a great deal about menopause, ageing, and that a calcium-rich diet can offset or help to prevent the onset of osteoporosis. It may come as a shock to many people that diets that are rich in animal-based proteins, and especially dairy products can actually help to give you osteoporosis and assist in its development. This is because that when digested, these products increase the pH balance of your blood. In other words, they produce a state where your blood becomes highly acidic.

Once the blood has become acid-rich, it must be neutralised before it causes damage to the infrastructure of the body. Normally, consuming enough vegetables and fruit will neutralise most of the acid if the right balance of foods has been consumed quickly enough. However, this is almost always never the case. Western diets are typically woefully inadequate in this respect and they cannot be relied upon to neutralise the acidic blood caused by dairy and meat protein consumption.

The body's next line of defence in neutralising acid blood is for the body to find another acid buffer. The most readily available acid-buffer for the body is calcium. Where does your body get the right source of readily available calcium? It cannot get any from the undigested dairy products. Your body naturally extracts it from your bones. Your body will dissolve your bones to produce enough alkaline to safely neutralise the high levels of acidic blood. It continues to do so until your blood pH balance reaches a tolerable level again. This mechanism is how milk and dairy foods can make your battle against osteoporosis much harder to manage and almost impossible to win.

My Next Steps

In summation of this section, menopause and all that it brings with it was not something that I was relishing the thought of enduring. As certain as night follows day, I could not avoid it unless I had a Dr Who TARDIS time machine to turn back my biological clock forever. The next logical question I had to answer, was what was I going to do about it? The key points of my quest I needed to address at all levels to either stop, reduce, slow down, minimise, or manage the effects of menopause were now as follows:

- ▲ I needed a high calcium diet that was not going to exasperate allergies, and/or stimulate cancer production etc.
- ▲ I should not consume excessive quantities of protein.
- ▲ I needed to perform weight-bearing resistance exercises to maintain and/or build maximum muscle while at the same time preventing or minimising osteoporosis.
- ▲ The exercises I needed to perform must be proven to be effective enough to do everything I wanted, while at the same time having the minimum stress impact effect on my body to prevent cortisol from causing weight/fat retention or gain.

The Overall Solution was Simple

- ▲ I should maintain my vegan diet.
- ▲ I should perform an isometric and a TRISOmetric™ exercise plan to deliver maximum stimulus with the minimum stress impact on my body and recovery system.
- ▲ I wanted a plan that anyone could perform, even as a complete beginner, and yet be able to add increasingly challenging but achievable layers as they progress and get stronger.
- ▲ I wanted a plan that would always provide an optimum workout for people at any level from absolute beginner right through to advanced athletes. The plans I devised and used are as follows:
  1. In order of difficulty, the most basic exercise plan would be to perform a single isometric exercise at roughly the mid-point along the ROM of the limb. Anyone could perform this routine, and if necessary, I could perform a minimum total-body workout in just 70 seconds of consecutive exercise time each day.
  2. The next level difficult up would be to perform an isometric exercise plan and to divide the Range Of Motion of each limb roughly equally into three parts. Then,

perform one isometric exercise in each position with no more than a 10-second rest between exercises.

3. The most advanced exercise plan, if I were advanced and fit enough to perform it, would be a TRISOmetric™ exercise plan. This would once again involve dividing the Range Of Motion of each limb roughly equally into three parts. Then, would perform one isometric exercise in each of those positions with no more than a 10-second rest between the exercises. Finally, and with only another 10-seconds of rest after the last isometric exercise, I would then perform a set of truly super-slow callisthenic (isotonic) exercises in super-strict style for a maximum of 3 repetitions.

In short, I needed to eat healthily, minimise, or limit any negative habits that would impede my progress, minimise stress where possible, get enough quality sleep, and then simply Muscle-up For Menopause!

Brain Fog

Before I move on to the sections about exercise science and the suggested exercises routines, no book on menopause would be complete without covering the dreaded issue of what is commonly called brain fog. This is one of the most frustrating things about menopause, and it is not commonly known or talked about.

Brain fog is an umbrella term for a memory function issue that can leave you annoyingly floundering to remember a word midsentence or the name of someone very familiar to you, you can often feel confused, concentrating on things can become a real issue, and multitasking skills you used to take for granted becomes much more challenging to harness.

Brian fog creeps up on you slowly as you approach menopause beginning with minor lapses in memory that are all too easily ignored and dismissed as being due to lack of sleep or too much prosecco during the previous weekend. One day, when you find yourself beginning your journey through full-blown menopause, brain fog can leave your embarrassingly struggling through life.

It is like all of a sudden someone has somehow removed your ability to make a rational decision about even the most basic of things. It is hard to focus your thoughts and even leave you fearful about showing signs of early-onset dementia. Unfortunately, over the years, many women have been misdiagnosed as having dementia syndrome or Alzheimer's disease when in fact they were actually suffering from menopausal brain fog instead. Women going through menopause and suffering from brain fog are more likely to have problems with increased symptoms of depression, they experience more hot flushes/flashes, more feelings of anxiety, and trouble sleeping.

When you are going through menopause and suffering brain fog, simple things can become big issues. For example, you can go to the kitchen to collect a couple of items as you rush to leave the house for a family day our and despite both items being right next to each other, somehow you can only see and focus on one of them to leave the other behind. You are not necessarily impaired and unable to function, even at work, it is more about having to consciously work harder to think clearly and function at your once typical base level. To add to the confusion for sufferers, the problem is typically all about short-term memory because long-term memory is almost always unaffected by this condition.

The good news is that menopause brain fog does not mean that you will say goodbye to your short-term memory forever because the effects are temporary. A four-year study found that post-menopause, there was a significant recovery in memory function. The research study was called "Effects of the menopause transition and hormone use on cognitive performance in midlife women" and was conducted by G A. Greendale, MD, M-H Huang, DrPh, R G. Wight, PhD, T Seeman, PhD, C Luetters, MS, N E. Avis, PhD, J Johnston, PhD, and A S. Karlamangla, PhD, MD.

Since menopause cannot be avoided, and therefore, a certain degree of brain fog will be experienced whether you like it or not, the most important question is, what can you do about it to help minimise the problem and the fallout that can surround it. Here are some of the practical approaches you can take to tackle both the symptoms of menopause and brain fog at the same time.

- Exercise regularly. We have established this already, and even if you are not going through menopause regular exercise has been shown to generally improve memory function. It also helps to promote better sleep at night and is a wonderful tool to help beat depression and feelings of anxiety.
- Adjust your diet. Again, we have already established the importance of diet for many reasons, and this is another good one to add to the list. Once again, it all comes back to minimising or better still eliminating all processed foods and only consuming natural unprocessed foods that are packed with nutrients. Naturally, and still surprising to many people, a vegan diet is the healthiest and best overall to help boost your memory function. I should also add that many women have benefited from what is commonly called the DASH diet (Dietary Approach to Stop Hypertension) and it is primarily designed to do exactly that. It could be worth exploring to help battle brain fog issues.
- Include soy protein in your diet. This is because some research has shown that supplementing your diet with soy isoflavone can have a positive effect on memory function. This was primarily in postmenopausal women, but there may also be benefits gained from this during menopause as well. I found out through experience and observation that when I have soy cream or soy milk in my coffee in the morning, my hot flushes/flashes are decreased during the day. If I skip this in the mornings, then my hot flashes can be an all-day rollercoaster of hot flushes/flashes followed by curious cold spells.
- Ensure that you are getting enough Vitamin B complex, and in particular, vitamin B12.

59

- ▲ Be careful not to spike your blood sugar levels with processed sugars from things like chocolate and sweets/candy.
- ▲ Try to maintain a good overall state of hydration which is good for all bodily functions, including the brain.
- ▲ Make more lists to help you remember things. Do not struggle, instead, embrace the situation as a temporary problem that you have to deal with, and making more use of lists to help you function will help with many things in life.
- ▲ Keep your mind active. This is good general advice anyway, but when facing menopause and the associated brain fog issues, it is worth taking even more seriously. Learning a new skill is a wonderful way to do this. Some people might choose computer/phone games, card games, volunteering to help at dog rescue centres as I/we do, painting, quilting, learning Tai Chi or another martial art that is both a mental challenge and a physical exercise combined. I learnt how to knit, and this has had a positive effect on my memory and ability to focus. It has also meant that both my husband and my greyhound dog now have almost every kind, colour, and type of knitted garment imaginable...

Chapter 3. Exercise Science Overview

In this section, we will give a user-friendly overview of exercise science together with the features and benefits of various exercise techniques and concepts. For those who want more in-depth information about the science of isometric exercise and health and fitness in general, then we suggest that you also read our books The ISOmetric Bible™ and The 70 Second Difference™ books. Both are available on Amazon.

The Basic Types of Resistance Exercise

All muscle training falls into between two or three specific categories, depending upon how you break them down. In the most basic form, there are two types, either contraction with movement, or contraction without movement. Breaking them down a step further there become three categories, with one being isotonic, another isokinetic. Last but certainly not least, is isometric.

Isotonic training is all about movement with muscle shortening and lengthening during the lifting and lowering phases of the exercise. We know that the isotonic category can be broken down further into three parts. One part is the concentric contraction, which is the lifting phase of an exercise when the muscles shorten in length. Another is the eccentric phase which is the lowering part of an exercise when the muscles lengthen.

Lastly in this isotonic category is the isokinetic contraction. This is where the muscle changes in length during both the concentric and eccentric phases of the contraction, however, the velocity remains constant no matter how much force is applied during the exercises.

Then comes the isometric category. With an isometric exercise, there is no movement whatsoever. To help you envision this, I will take a random weight training or freehand callisthenic exercise such as a chest press because it can be performed either with movement OR without movement, as an isometric exercise.

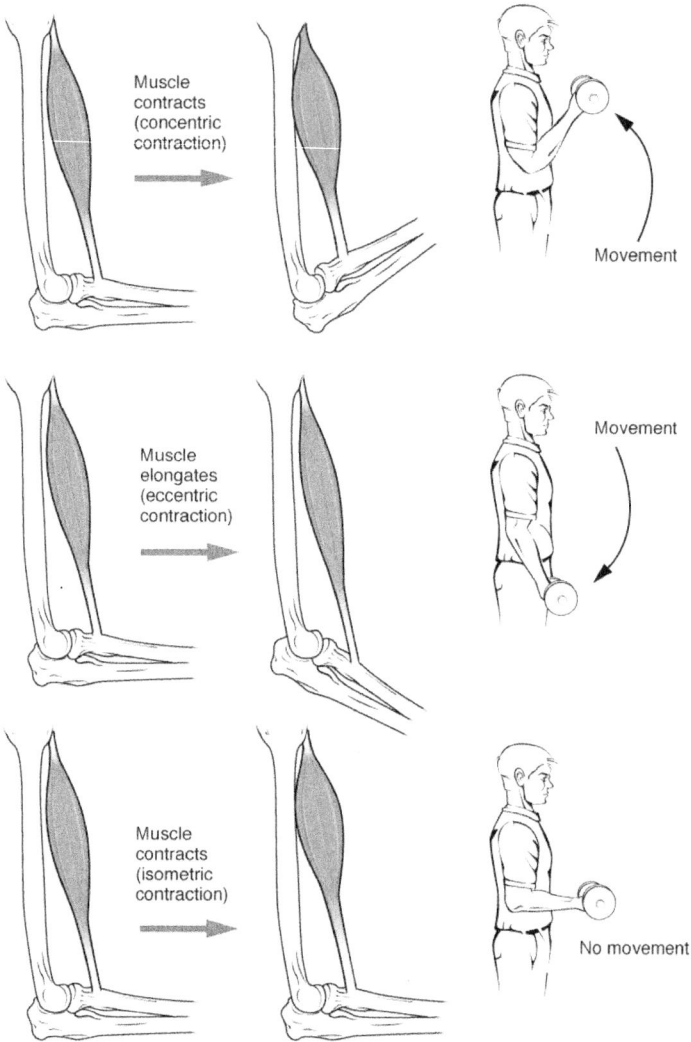

Basic Types of Contraction in Resistance Exercise-picture credit OpenStax

For example, a barbell, a machine, or your bodyweight can be lifted and lowered to perform an exercise such as a barbell curl, this is called, isotonic exercise, callisthenics or simply exercise with movement.

To perform the same or similar exercise isometrically you would attempt to perform the same or similar biomechanically correct actions of a barbell curl, however, at a certain point, or points if multiple exercise points were being used, the curling movement would stop because an immovable object point had been reached.

At that point or points, you would apply an increasing level of intensity until you reach the desired target level as you attempt to perform the curling exercise against the immovable object.

At the desired isometric exercise point, a constant force is applied against the immovable object for 7 seconds which is the optimum isometric exercise time. The ideal basic isometric exercise point for general exercise is roughly at the mid-point when your muscles reach a stalemate working against each other or an immovable object. This is called a Standard isometric Contraction.

The harder you engage your muscles as you try to break the stalemate by lifting, pushing, or pulling, then the stronger your muscles become. In doing so, you engage many more muscle fibres than normal as you attempt to move the immovable object and perform the curling exercise action.

Doors, desks, chairs, walls, and many other everyday items work well as immovable objects BUT the easiest and most used immovable object is typically yourself.

Isometric Overview

As you now know, isometric exercise does not involve any movement. Instead, the joint angle and the muscle length do not change during contraction. You also now know that 7 seconds is now regarded as the optimum time to perform an isometric exercise.

Almost everyone when exercising tends to count the exercise elapsed time much faster than real elapsed time. This means that it is easy not to reach the magic 7 seconds of the optimum isometric exercise time. Therefore, we always suggest aiming to perform the exercise for 10 seconds to ensure that the 7-second target is always reached even when under the stress of performing intense exercise.

Isometric exercise has been extensively scientifically researched and has been proven repeatedly to be a highly efficient way to build great strength and grow muscle. In fact, isometric exercise is probably one of the most thoroughly researched of all exercise systems. It also remains one of the most misunderstood systems of exercise.

Several different techniques can be used in the isometric exercise system. Most of these techniques are highly advanced for use by competitive athletes, competitive martial arts practitioners, strength athletes and bodybuilders. They have no application as part of a general isometric exercise session for the average person who simply wants to get generally stronger and fitter.

Purely out of interest I will list them here, and in case any fitness enthusiast, athletes or bodybuilders read this book and wish to try them. They are described in greater detail in our book called The Isometric Bible which is available on Amazon and good bookstores. The most common and advanced isometric exercise techniques include the following:

- △ Standard Isometric Contraction
- △ Yielding Isometric Contraction
- △ Maximum Duration Isometrics
- △ Oscillatory Isometrics
- △ Impact Absorption Isometrics
- △ Explosive Isometrics, AKA: Ballistic Isometrics
- △ Static-Dynamic Isometric
- △ Isometric Contrast
- △ Functional Isometrics
- △ TRISOmetrics™

There are more than enough isometric exercises that can be performed without any equipment whatsoever to allow a total body workout routine to be completed relatively easily. These will typically be self-resisted isometric exercises, which are excellent. By using only minimal readily available equipment such as walking poles, golf clubs, martial arts belts, climbing ropes, scuba diving webbing weight belts, and broom handles etc. it is possible to greatly expand the number of exercises that can be performed.

It is also perfectly possible to adapt and use other readily available items such as tow ropes, steel chains, towels, and commonly found immobile objects such as sturdy fixed barrier railings, solid walls, solid doors, door frames, or parked vehicles to perform a complete isometric exercise routine. Again, these are all excellent improvised exercise tools that allow an expanded range of highly effective isometric exercises to be performed.

Using improvised exercise tools can yield an unexpected additional benefit. This is that it allows one to focus more and apply greater concentration to each exercise. This is particularly useful for those who are either completely new to, or who are relatively new to the isometric exercise system. We will explain more about what these can be later in the book.

One of the things we love about both the isometric and self-resisted system of exercise is that as you get stronger through exercise, then you can apply more force and intensity to your isometric or self-resisted exercises.

This means that you can gradually increase the level of intensity you can safely apply to each exercise which will mean that the results and benefits you receive will grow in a compound way through regular daily use. This is what we call a natural Adaptive Response™ mechanism which is a useful aspect of our biology.

Isometric Exercise Science

Even until the mid-20th century, there was almost no scientific research that had been performed into the benefits of isometric exercise. We also know that before the first serious scientific research study, how people trained isometrically was typically by performing what we now call endurance isometrics. Thankfully, isometric exercise has now been thoroughly scientifically researched and proven for several decades. I would estimate that there has probably been at least as much scientific research performed into isometric exercise as there has been into traditional resistance training.

The first major in-depth study into isometric exercise was performed at the world-famous Max Plank Institute in Dortmund, Germany. If you already have a reasonable knowledge of science, you will also know that the Max Plank Institute is a world-renowned centre of scientific excellence in many disciplines.

Between 1953 and 1958, one of the most extensive research studies was commissioned into isometric exercise science. These experiments are now considered by many to be the original gold standard of isometric exercise studies. The results were made widespread public knowledge in the resultant ground-breaking book, The Physiology of Strength, by Dr Theodor Hettinger - Research Fellow at the Max Plank Institute. During that 5-year research period, Dr Hettinger and Dr Muller performed a widely reported, reputed 5,500 experiments, although this figure is almost certainly apocryphal because they would have had to perform a minimum of three experiments a day, every day for five years. Research suggests that the actual number of experiments performed by Hettinger and Muller was probably closer to 200, however, in wider studies at other institutions since that time, over 5,500 studies have almost certainly been completed. These were conducted on male and female volunteers from all walks of life, and at every level of strength, fitness, and athletic ability. Perhaps what surprised people the most was how dramatic and impressive the results were gained from performing isometric exercises. Also, because the same or similar results were easily repeatable it made the data gained from the experiments exceptionally reliable.

The conclusion of the extensive studies proved beyond doubt the overall superiority of isometric exercise when it comes to building both strength and muscle, compared to traditional isotonic exercises methods. It also proved that the isometric system delivered these results much faster and with far less exercise than through traditional resistance training.

Another extremely interesting result emerged from the experiments. This was that it was not the length of time that an isometric exercise was held that produced the optimum results. Instead, it was the correct level of intensity applied for a very specific optimum time.

They found that by performing only one daily isometric exercise for between only 6 and 7 seconds, and at only two-thirds of an individual's maximum effort, it could increase strength by an average of up to 5% per week. By any standards, strength gains of 5% in exchange for the expenditure of only 66%, or around two-thirds of an individual's maximum capacity, is an excellent result.

Perhaps even more amazingly, they discovered that after someone has performed a single 7-second training stimulus (exercise) per day, the muscle being exercised in that same position was no longer responsive to further gains. In other words, it did not matter how many more times you exercised the same muscle in the same position, there would be no further increase in muscle growth or strength. The only way to do this was to perform another isometric exercise at a different position only the ROM (Range Of Motion) of the limb being exercised. The scientific data about this can be referenced on pages 28 to 31 of Dr Theodor Hettinger's book, "The Physiology of Strength."

In 2001, Nicolas Babault PhD of the University of Burgundy, Dijon, France, led a team of scientists to research and examine how many muscle fibres were activated, and how long they remained active during both traditional weight training and isometric training.

(*The scientific research paper is published: Nicolas Babault, Michel Pousson, Yves Ballay, and Jacques Van Hoecke - Groupe Analyse du Mouvement, Unite´ de Formation et de Recherche Sciences et Techniques des Activite's Physiques et Sportives, Universite' de Bourgogne, BP 27877, 21078 Dijon Cedex, France.)*

They discovered that when training intensely, and in near-perfect style, the levels of muscle activation during repetitions of optimum maximal weight training were between 89.7% during the concentric contraction, or when lifting a weight, and 88.3% during the eccentric contraction, or when lowering a weight. For practical purposes, an average of about 89% overall.

The study also revealed that during the lifting, or concentric part of the exercise, the maximum intramuscular tension only lasted for between 0.25 and 0.5 seconds. Which, for practical purposes is an average of about 1/3rd of a second during each isotonic repetition.

This is because traditional isotonic resistance exercises naturally involve movement. They also have aspects of velocity and acceleration to consider in the overall equation. "Force" is only produced for a split second, to produce a maximal contraction of the muscle fibres.

The same research also showed that the level of muscle activation during isometric exercise was as high as 95.2% and that it lasted for the entire 7 to 10 seconds of each exercise. This is a huge increase over the 1/3rd of second muscular activation achieved during a single repetition of weight training.

Based on these discoveries, then technically a single isometric exercise performed at only two-thirds of an individual's overall maximum can deliver either similar or often even better results, than the equivalent of up to 3 sets of 10 weight training repetitions in the lifting phase of the exercise.

To explain this further I will use a typical barbell curl exercise in the lifting phase as my example, where the object of the exercise is to engage as many muscle fibres as possible in a maximum muscular contraction. Naturally, 3 sets of 10 repetitions give us an overall total of 30 repetitions. One set of 10 repetitions of the barbell curl in perfect high-intensity style produces a total maximum muscular engagement for a total of approximately 3.3 seconds. Three sets of 10 repetitions of the same exercise, a total of 30 repetitions will result in a total of approximately 9.9 seconds of maximum muscular engagement, and an average of 89% muscle activation overall.

In comparison, if one high-intensity isometric contraction exercise produces a maximum muscular engagement that lasts for the entire duration of the exercise. Even though the optimum time over which an isometric exercise is performed was found to be 7 seconds, this is almost always rounded up to the 10-second target number. The maximum muscular engagement will last for the entire 10 seconds of a high-intensity isometric exercise and with 95.2% muscle activation overall.

This is proof that is based entirely on scientific research that 3 sets of 10 near-perfect high-intensity curls when weight training, which takes several minutes to perform, still was not equal to the results achieved by a single 10-second high-intensity isometric curl exercise.

The Standard Isometric Contraction

The standard isometric contraction is a simple and highly effective technique. This is the technique we will focus on for practical isometric training.

The standard isometric contraction, AKA: overcoming isometric contraction, AKA: maximum-effort isometrics, or whatever else you wish to call it, is when a muscle is applying force to push or pull against an immovable resistance. This is the most basic of all kinds of isometric exercise, and it is highly effective.

This type of isometric contraction exercise was performed during the experiments by Dr T. Hettinger and Dr E. Muller at the Max Plank Institute. It is also the technique referred to in their book "The Physiology of Strength."

In a standard isometric contraction, it is theoretically possible to exert up to 100% of one's maximum capacity effort against an immovable object and then continue to hold that level of intensity throughout the exercise. This means that standard isometric contraction can be a very high-intensity exercise system.

Performing an isometric exercise against an immovable object at a certain level of intensity for a given duration of time will teach your body to recruit more muscle fibres to try to move the object. As you perform the exercise and generate as much force as possible, your CNS, or Central Nervous System, learns that it needs to activate and recruit more muscle fibres to reach the goal of moving the object.

Since this will naturally be impossible to move, the process will continue each time you exercise to make you stronger and grow more muscle. Your body mechanisms become trained to readily activate and recruit additional muscle fibres as needed when facing repeated similar challenges, which in turn, repeats the cycle more readily every time.

As we mentioned earlier, the immovable/solid object that is used can be anything that is completely solid and completely safe to use. This can be a wall, a door, door jamb, parked motor vehicle or anything similar. Perhaps the most common objects used to enhance everyday isometric exercise training are sturdy towels, climbing rope, martial arts belts, scuba diving weight belts, webbing straps, golf clubs, and broom handles, etc. All the aforementioned items are excellent when used properly, and all will deliver some excellent results. More importantly, they are typically readily available for most people which makes exercising with them so much easier.

Another common way to perform isometric exercise is to do it in a self-resisted way. Self-resisted means that you push or pull against your limbs, hands, and feet, etc.

For example, you might place the palms of your hands together at chest level with your hands roughly at the midpoint of your body. In that position, you would then press your hands together using your chest muscles to provide the primary driving force. Suddenly, you are performing a highly effective self-resisted isometric chest exercise!

It is possible to perform a well-balanced and highly effective self-resisted isometric workout to exercise virtually every section of the body. So, never underestimate self-resisted exercise because it can be immensely powerful indeed. Also, self-resistance exercises are an excellent way to ensure that a personal maximum resistance is used safely, and with minimum risk of injury caused by applying too much force.

The fact is that it does not matter which method is chosen. It can be isometrics performed against an immovable object, self-resisted isometrics, or a combination of the two. The most important thing is that either the object must be completely immovable through human muscle power alone, or the force of one body part must be able to completely counterbalance the force of another body part to produce a muscular stalemate.

Workout Intensity

Intensity is always going to be a relative term, and it is often completely misunderstood when it is used concerning exercise. When it comes to exercising your muscles, the intensity is the % of your ability to move a resistance. Technically, an individual's highest possible level of intensity is when they reach a point of momentary failure after exerting themselves completely.

However, the important questions we need to try and find answers to are: "How hard is hard?" and "How intense is intense?" To some degree, both are very subjective things. Taking two people of roughly equal fitness, something that is intense to one person might be considered comparatively easy to the other.

Hard is a relative term, and handling 50 lbs of resistance is impossibly hard if your strength is only at the level required to lift 49 lbs. However, if you can lift 100 lbs as a maximum, then lifting 50 lbs is going to be comparatively easy.

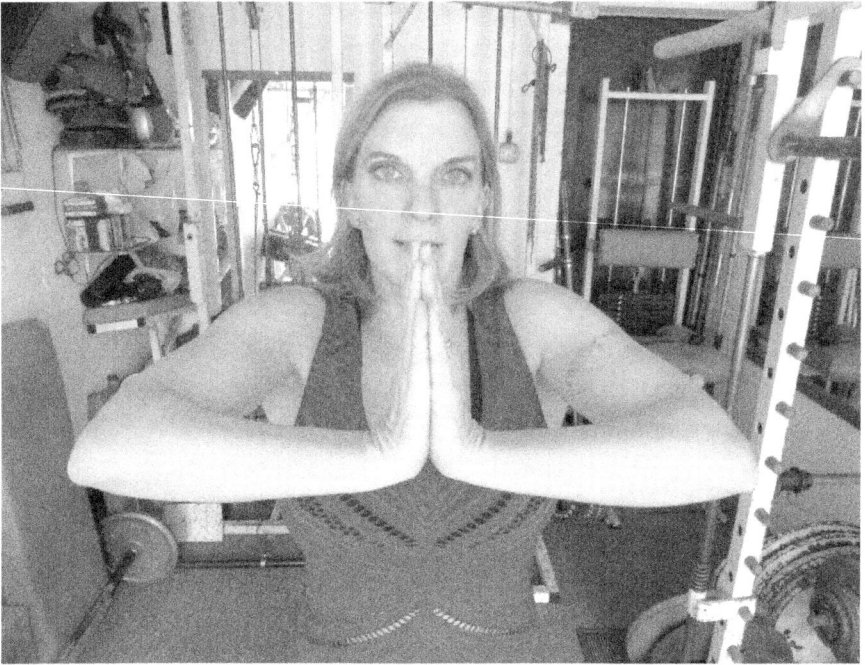

Often, the only factors differentiating between people and the intensity level exerted, are going to be mental toughness, determination, and perception.

Therefore, to gain the greatest benefits from isometric exercise the first thing that must be learned is how to determine, with a reasonable degree of accuracy, what level of intensity is being applied to an exercise.

It is just a fact that what one person deems to be 100% of their capacity will always be quite different from another person's estimate. The accurate estimation of what one person deems to be 2/3^{rds} of their overall maximum intensity will also vary from person to person. The accuracy of estimation will also vary greatly between an experienced professional athlete and an absolute beginner to exercise.

Experience has taught us that most people who are new to exercise will always fall well short of accurate estimation of any given percentage. A beginner will find it more challenging to accurately estimate what 2/3^{rds} of their 100% maximum is when compared to a more experienced athlete. Many people might believe that they are performing at 100% capacity when they are only performing at around only 2/3^{rds}, or even perhaps at only 50% or less of their 100% maximum.

This is because exercise is new to them, therefore, the experiences and feelings in their body which are associated with it are also new. They simply have no common frame of reference when it comes to calculating/estimating their level of physical exertion.

The human brain has a built-in mechanism that helps to protect the body and prevent it from performing a physical activity to such a level that could cause serious damage or even death. This is the mechanism that makes your brain tell you to stop exercising when it begins to get tough, and the feeling of wanting to stop exercising only increases as you continue to push yourself harder to do more. This is all despite the biological fact that you are physically capable of doing much more than is being suggested by the messages you are receiving from yourself.

Over time, the brain of people who exercise regularly, and especially to a high level of intensity, will naturally adjust, and reposition this built-in safety margin. This means that the brain of an experienced high-level athlete does not "tell" them to stop an exercise until the level of intensity is much higher than it would be for a beginner.

Therefore, when it comes to exercise, how is it possible to subjectively quantify, and then impart appropriate levels of recommended intensity?   This problem is made even more challenging when one considers the fact that accurately translating and subjectively assessing various levels of intensity will, to some degree, always be subjective to every individual.

If you were to train as hard as humanly possible, with near 100% maximum intensity which involves super-strict form, and training to complete failure and beyond, then you simply cannot train for a long time. It is just physiologically impossible. Physics and biology are quite simple in this respect.

The intensity of your workout is directly proportional to the length of time that you are physically able to perform your workout. The harder and more intensely you exercise, then the shorter time that you will be physically able to perform the exercise.

Make no mistake, performing a 7-second isometric exercise while exerting close to your personal 100% maximum physical capacity is completely and utterly exhausting, even for a professional athlete.

What does all this mean when it comes to accurately communicating various levels of exercise intensity, especially when there is no professional coach or elaborate and expensive measuring equipment at hand?

Research clearly shows that almost everyone will stop exercising long before they are in any danger of becoming seriously fatigued. Most people will *think* they are achieving a much higher level of intensity than they would do if they were only a little more mentally resilient.

This does not mean that people should suddenly begin pushing themselves beyond their physical limits, which would be a stupid thing to do. However, it does mean that most people who enjoy a higher than average level of mental resilience and determination, as well as being in physically good condition, can push themselves much harder than they might think. If anyone ever feels "genuine" strain or fatigue to the point of becoming injured, then they should stop exercising immediately.

Even without the aid of a professional coach to monitor, encourage you and measure your intensity and progress with specialist equipment, the tips we have outlined in this section will help you to get the most out of every workout. It is also worth remembering that if you cheat, then the only person who loses is "you."

Technically, How Does a Muscle Grow?

How does a muscle grow? This is one of the most common questions asked concerning fitness and exercise in general. It is also one of the most misunderstood concepts, even amongst fitness professionals and personal trainers. To see for yourself just how uninformed or badly informed some people are, simply join one or two of the social media groups online so you can read some of the absolute drivel posted by 'keyboard warriors' who purport to be 'experts' on the subject. Alarmingly, many of these people seem to have developed a hardcore following, which to the science-based professional is like watching 'fools leading other fools' on a wild goose chase.

Back to the key question which is, how does a muscle grow? To explain this, we must examine three concepts, which are: 1) muscle growth through increases in the volume/size of myofibrils inside the muscles, which is commonly termed as being myofibrillar hypertrophy. 2) hyperplasia, which is when there is an increase in the number of muscle cells/fibres. 3) sarcoplasmic growth which is all about increasing the fluid content.

When it comes to the subject of exercise, the muscles you wish to grow must be challenged with a workload that is greater than they can currently accommodate. In other words, exercise that is intense enough to stimulate growth. This stimulus can come from any source such as lifting a heavy object, weight training, isometrics, through compressing a spring in a device such as a Bullworker™, or through self-resistance either hand to hand / limb to limb / using an Iso-Bow™ etc.

This process creates trauma to the muscle fibres which disrupts the muscle cell organelles. This then triggers other cells outside the muscle fibres to greatly increase in numbers at and around the point of the trauma to repair the damage. The process of repair involves a fusion of cells.

This, in turn, causes the cross-sectional area of the muscle fibre to increase because the muscle cell myofibrils increase in both size and quantity. This process is more commonly known as hypertrophy. Since this process increases the number of cellular nuclei the muscle fibres generate more myosin and actin. These are contractile protein myofilaments which in turn help to make the muscle stronger.

This is the basis of what is more commonly known as myofibril muscle growth. In addition to this, there is also probably a process called hyperplasia which takes place. I use the term, 'probably' because this concept is extremely controversial for many reasons. One of the key problems is that evidence of this in human beings is lacking, whereas there is a mass of evidence supporting hyperplasia in mice and other animals.

Hypertrophy is the increase in the size of the existing muscle fibres to accommodate the increased demands placed upon them through intense exercise. Hyperplasia, concerning skeletal muscle growth, is the increase in the number of muscle fibres which in turn will also increase the cross-sectional area of a muscle.

Despite there being a lack of evidence supporting hyperplasia in human beings, logic supports the process taking place. This is because of a theory known as Nuclear Domain Theory. This states that the nucleus of a cell (a muscle cell in this instance) is only able to control a finite area of cellular space. It is thought that satellite cells donate their nuclei to the muscle cell until a certain point is reached whereby this can no longer take place.

Beyond a certain limit, and through continued intense training, the cell must eventually divide to create two cells instead of the former single cell. When this happens, the entire hypertrophy process starts over once again. This probably means that most of the muscle growth is almost certainly caused by hypertrophy, and a much smaller percentage can be attributed to hyperplasia at any given point in the muscle stimulus/growth process.

There is a subject of sarcoplasmic muscle growth to address. Sarcoplasmic muscle growth is the increase in the volume of sarcoplasmic fluid in the muscle cell. These are the fluid and energy resources surrounding the myofibrils in your muscles containing mostly glycogen together with other elements including creatine, ATP, and water etc.

To clarify, glycogen is simply a type of sugar that serves as a form of energy. It is deposited in bodily tissues as a store of carbohydrates, and it is the body's main form of storage for the sugar, glucose. Glycogen is stored in two main places in the body, one being the liver, and the other being the muscles.

Glycogen is the body's secondary source of long-term energy storage, with the primary energy storage source being fat. When glycogen is in the muscles, it is converted into glucose for use as energy when performing sports etc., and glycogen stored in the liver is converted into glucose for use as energy throughout the body, and in the central nervous system.

Sarcoplasmic growth increases the muscle volume, but this increase is not in functional strength mass since it does not increase the number of muscle fibres. It is like 'the pump,' in that it is an increase in the size and shape of the muscle through the muscle holding an increased amount of fluid.

Rest Time Between Exercises

The rest time taken between exercises during a workout is quite different from the rest and recovery needed to recover and allow your body to positively respond to the stimulus generated by exercise.

If you keep the rest time between exercises brief enough, then the workout routine itself will give you an excellent cardiovascular workout, and this is what we recommend that you ultimately aim for. If you are already very fit, then we would recommend that instead of performing the optional cardio routine, and you simply put more effort and intensity into each isometric exercise.

At the same time, aim to keep the rest time between those exercises as brief as possible. This approach will help you work towards being able to perform each exercise so that it has an Ultra-High Intensity

Ultra-Short Burst™ effect, which will greatly improve your overall fitness level, and boost your Base Metabolic Rate or BMR.

If you are not already fit, then to begin with you may wish to simply allow each isometric exercise to deliver all the cardio you need as you gradually build up your levels of fitness and endurance. Eventually, you will soon increase your level of fitness to a point where you can begin to gradually reduce the rest time between each exercise to a minimum point that works best for you.

Once you have learned how to fully engage the muscles during each exercise with sufficient intensity, and at the same time, you have learned how to breathe fully, deeply, and naturally throughout each exercise. At the same time, you should be keeping the rest time between exercises to a minimum because this combination will have an excellent and beneficial cardiovascular effect.

Dynamic Flexation™

Dynamic Flexation™ is a technique we devised to help ensure that we gained maximum benefit from the isometric portion of our exercise regimens. I will recap and briefly summarise the Dynamic Flexation™ technique as originally laid out in "The 70 Second Difference™" book.

We always recommend that everyone who performs any kind of resistance exercise practices some form of Dynamic Flexation™ before performing any exercise. This will help to ensure that all muscles, tendons, ligaments, joints, and your spine have become naturally and properly engaged in the correct biomechanical exercise position.

We would never recommend that as soon as you assume any exercise position that you suddenly apply maximum power and intensity right away. This is unless you are a very experienced athlete, or unless you are training with a qualified coach to perform a certain type of isometric exercise to develop extra power such as a static-dynamic or explosive/ballistic isometric technique. Instead, we recommend that you always breathe naturally as you gradually flex and engage your muscles and joints into performing the exercise.

To perform Dynamic Flexation™ you gradually flex your grip and the muscles you are about to exercise while applying an increasing level of intensity immediately before performing the exercise. The exercise is then performed, and to disengage from the exercise we recommend reversing the Dynamic Flexation™ engagement process.

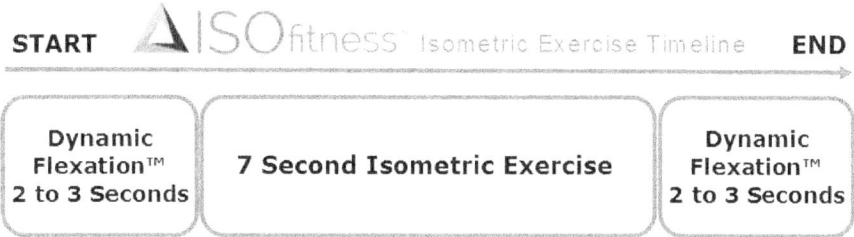

START ◢ISO‌fitness™ Isometric Exercise Timeline **END**

Dynamic Flexation™ 2 to 3 Seconds	7 Second Isometric Exercise	Dynamic Flexation™ 2 to 3 Seconds

Our preference is to apply tension and intensity to the exercise gradually through Dynamic Flexation™ typically for between 2 and 3 seconds, or even for as long as 4 seconds if needed. This all takes place before beginning to count the required 7-second exercise time of the isometric contraction.

We prefer using one deep full breath in and out as a method of more accurately counting each second that has elapsed. This way, you will time each exercise more accurately, and you will not be tempted to hold your breath at any point which is a mistake that beginners often make.

Similarly, at the end of an exercise, we do not recommend that it be ended abruptly. Instead, we recommend reversing the Dynamic Flexation™ technique so that you gradually relax as you slightly move each muscle and joint out of the exercise position.

This process helps enormously because when you are in an advantageous position it will help you to gain the maximum benefit from each exercise you perform. Dynamic Flexation™ is when you move and adjust either your feet, legs/leg, hips and especially your hands as you gradually assume a solid position and handgrip. As you flex and move, you will be making micro-adjustments.

79

All exercises will be performed best if you assume a correct and solid handgrip, fist clench, or foot position etc. One of the most important aspects of assuming the correct exercise position begins with your grip. Without a solid grip on a bar, handle, or anything else you need to hold while exercising, you will naturally be setting yourself up to perform sub-maximally. You can also be helping to develop injuries which can include sore elbows, joints, ligaments, and tendons.

Dynamic Flexation™ is a concept that embraces the broader principles of motor unit recruitment, and "Henneman's Size Principle" to increase the contractile strength of a muscle. Elwood Henneman's principle stated that under load, the motor units in a muscle are engaged according to their magnitude of force output, from the smallest to the largest, and in task-appropriate order.

This means that the slow-twitch, low-force, fatigue-resistant muscle fibres are activated before any fast-twitch, high-force muscle fibres are engaged which are less fatigue-resistant. Since the body naturally works in this way, it enables precise and finely controlled force to be delivered at all levels of output.

This also means that when exercising, or when performing tasks in daily life, the fatigue which is experienced as a result will always be minimised. It will also be proportional to the sequential engagement of the most appropriate muscle fibres being engaged.

Isometric Exercises and Blood Pressure

Some exercise critics point out the fact that when someone performs an isometric exercise it will raise their blood pressure. However, the same people also very conveniently forget that the same is also true of all other forms of exercise including freehand callisthenics and traditional isotonic resistance training with weights.

ALL physical activity, and especially exercise will cause your blood pressure to rise for a short time. Providing that you are in good health, that you always breathe deeply, naturally, and normally when performing any exercise, then any rise in blood pressure will soon return to a normal level when the exercise is stopped. The faster this happens, the fitter you are.

For those who are advanced athletes and/or are used to hard and intense isometric training for a long time, then you will already have made significant progress in strengthening your heart and circulatory system.

For those who are new to isometric training, just like with any form of exercise, the best way into it is by taking it slowly and less intensely at first.

Newcomers to exercise, and especially isometrics, should always focus on applying less intensity, to begin with, and on always breathing fully and deeply throughout all exercises. NEVER HOLD YOUR BREATH!

Under strict medical supervision, even those with Coronary Artery Disease and high blood pressure should be able to increase their physical activity levels with a reasonable degree of safety safely. However, if you are a person who already suffers from high blood pressure, then you should always exercise at a much lower level of intensity than someone who has no physical issues.

Furthermore, **EVERYONE, AND ESPECIALLY PEOPLE WITH HYPERTENSION, OR ANY FORM OF CARDIOVASCULAR DISEASE, SHOULD ALWAYS CHECK WITH THEIR DOCTOR BEFORE BEGINNING ANY KIND OF EXERCISE ROUTINE**.

Rest and Recovery

When calculating your ideal recovery period, many things must be taken into consideration. These include your age, your current health and fitness level, the quantity of exercise taken, and most importantly the intensity of the exercise which has been performed.

Some people will need a recovery period of between 24 and 48 hours, and for others, the recovery period may be as brief as between 12 and 24 hours.

As a rule, the recovery period will always incrementally increase as the intensity of the exercises increases towards an individual's 100% potential maximum capacity. Always be aware of this and make sure that you factor this into your rest and recovery time calculations. The diagram will help to outline this.

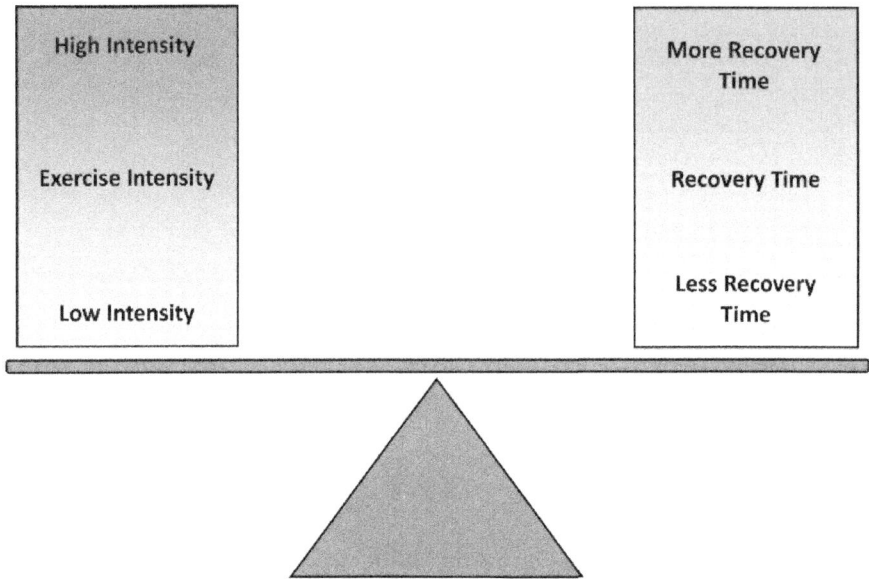

Sports scientist J. Atha's research revealed something remarkable. This was that when performing isometric contraction exercises at two-thirds of an individual's maximum capacity, the average person could safely perform an exercise like this daily, without overtraining.

Standard isometric contraction exercises can be safely performed daily, by almost anyone, of almost any age, and in almost any physical condition as a means of strength development, body shaping, and even for bodybuilding.

For more intense workouts, then we recommend a full rest day between workouts due to the higher demands being placed upon the Central Nervous System (CNS) and the time needed to fully recover and benefit from the exercise.

Several other factors affect post-exercise recovery. These include a balanced and properly executed stretching routine and getting enough quality sleep. While you sleep, your body releases certain hormones which help you to repair and rebuild damaged tissue, and which will directly help your muscles to grow.

Adequate Nutrition is Vital

Post-exercise high-quality nutrition will help your body to repair itself faster, decrease your recovery time, and will help to generally maximise the benefits gained from the exercise. Studies indicate that there is a 30 to 60-minute time window after exercise when you need to eat, and after which, your body begins to draw upon itself to repair and recover from your exercise session. Drinking enough water is also one of the most important factors in your recovery process, as well as for overall health. This is because your muscles are mostly composed of water.

Since research has shown that post-exercise immunodepression peaks if one exercises for longer than we are technically naturally physically able this becomes an even bigger problem if this scenario is further enhanced due to reduced or inadequate food intake.

The availability of certain key nutrients is vital when recovering from heavy exercise to ensure a robust immune system is maintained and there are enough resources to build muscle. Most people mistakenly consume excessive amounts of protein at the expense of other key nutrients such as carbohydrates. In doing this they are working against their best interests and overall optimum health.

One of the key nutrients that help the body recover from prolonged periods of heavy exercise is carbohydrates. There is a lot of research supporting the hypothesis that carbohydrate is the most important nutritional factor in preventing post-exercise immunodepression. People either conveniently forget or are completely ignorant of the fact that the protein composition of human muscle is typically only somewhere in the region of between 18% and 21% protein and the rest is made up of water, glucose, lipids, and carbohydrates etc.

We will not go into extensive detail here in this section of the book, however, if you want to learn more about this and many other surprising nuggets of useful information about nutrition and exercise then they can be found in The 70 Second Difference book.

Strength, Stamina, Endurance, and Resilience

It is important to understand the difference between strength, stamina and endurance because once understood, you will then be able to devise the most suitable workout routines according to your body type.

Muscular strength is possibly best understood as being a muscle's capacity to exert force against resistance, or weight. This is comparatively easy to measure because your ability to lift a given amount of weight for a single repetition is a good measure of your strength.

Stamina is the length of time at which a muscle, or group of muscles, can perform at or near your maximum capacity. For example, the number of squats you can perform with a given weight which is 90% of your maximum would be a measure of your stamina or the overall distance that you can carry a similarly heavy object such as an anvil.

Endurance is all about time, and your ability to perform a certain muscular action for a prolonged period regardless of the capacity at which you are working.

Resilience is all about your ability to recover from whatever stresses and demands are placed upon your muscles. However, resilience is mostly all about your state of mind, your mental toughness and ability to endure, perform and deliver under pressure, and about how you recover quickly emotionally.

The muscular composition of your body will always determine how well you will perform in certain sports. The amount of slow twitch muscle fibres you possess will determine how well you perform at endurance-related events, and both type A and type B fast twitch muscle fibres are all about explosive power and your ability to maintain it.

In simple terms, if you possess mostly slow twitch fibres, then you are naturally going to be better suited to endurance sports. Alternatively, if you possess mostly fast twitch muscle fibres, then you are a natural weightlifter. It is important to note, that no matter what your natural predisposition might be in this respect, with the correct training regimen, it is still possible to significantly increase your abilities in your naturally weaker opposing areas of speciality.

The TRISOmetric™ Exercise Concept

The TRISOmetric™ exercise concept was first developed in the mid-1980s by Brian Sterling-Vete PhD as a high-intensity method when he was training with 4-times World's Strongest Man Jon Pall Sigmarsson in Iceland. He wanted to dramatically increase the training intensity without simply increasing the weight we were lifting and reducing the rest time between. Then weight increases would follow at the newly elevated level of base intensity.

The TRISOmetric™ exercise can be performed with any type of resistance equipment, however, it equally does not necessarily need a gym or gym equipment in order to get a good workout session. It is perfectly possible, and to many people preferable, to perform a TRISOmetric™ exercise workout using self-resisted isometric exercises or a range of simple IIEDs or Improvised Isometric Exercise Devices.

These can comprise readily available items such as climbing rope, a doorway pull-up bar, or a towel. The TRISOmetric™ exercise technique can also be performed very easily with a Bullworker®, Steel Bow®, Iso-Bow®, and/or Iso-Gym®, or a combination of all the above. The Iso-Bow® is our preferred exercise device of choice, preferably a pair of them.

The TRISOmetric™ exercise system is a combination of three scientifically proven techniques into a single unified approach. These are as follows.

- ▲ Level 1 – Single Position Isometric Exercise.
    - o Isometric exercise is proven to be more efficient at building strength and muscle than traditional isotonic exercise.
- ▲ Level 2 – Triple Position Isometric Exercises.
    - o Dividing the ROM (Range Of Motion) into three segment points of roughly equal distance, and then performing an isometric exercise at each point, will deliver even muscle building and strength gains across the entire ROM of the limb being exercised.
- ▲ Level 3 – Combine Super-Slow Isotonic Exercise with level 2.
    - o Super-slow isotonic exercise delivers better gains in muscle size and strength than by performing the same exercise faster. Super-slow exercises engage more muscle fibres for longer.

The system also incorporates other scientifically proven aspects including a specific length of time taken between each exercise, and Ultra Short Ultra High-intensity bursts of exercise etc. Since isometric exercise is one of the most efficient and result-producing in terms of the ratio of the effort expended and results gained.

In practice, to perform one complete set of a TRISOmetric™ exercise, firstly, a single isometric exercise is performed in each of three positions along the ROM (Range Of Motion) of the body part being exercised. Each of the isometric positions chosen will divide the range of motion of the limb roughly into three equal parts. This way a more even strength curve is developed for the muscle being exercised. This takes advantage of the strength gain overlap area of + and – 20% around the point of isometric exercise chosen. However, more equally divided isometric exercise positions can be employed by more advanced practitioners.

Next, the focus is on rest time. There must be no longer than 10 seconds of rest time between each isometric exercise. Once all three (or more) isometric exercises have been completed, then once again with a maximum rest time of just 10 seconds, an appropriate isotonic exercise is performed to exercise the same muscles or muscle group. The isotonic exercise can be performed with either a Bullworker®, a Steel Bow®, an Iso-Bow®, and Iso-gym®, as freehand callisthenics or with weights/resistance machines.

It really does not matter what equipment you use, or if you use any equipment, or not. The correct execution of the corresponding exercise is what is most important. The isotonic portion should be performed in super-slow style. This means that each repetition should take 10 to 12 seconds to perform in the concentric or lifting phase where the muscles shorten, and another 10 to 12 seconds to perform in the eccentric or lowering phase where the muscles lengthen.

If you perform each portion of the TRISOmetric™ exercise correctly, then you will find it extremely intense. We recommend that you do not attempt to repeat the exercise again and that you do not perform any other exercise for the same muscle/muscle group. The fact is that if you perform the TRISOmetric™ exercise correctly you will probably NOT be able to or indeed have any desire to perform more. it is all about focus, intensity, and the quality of what you do, and jot about the quantity.

During the experimental phase as I developed the TRISOmetric™ exercise concept, I concluded that it was better for the CNS, or Central Nervous System, to perform the isometric phases first. The data I gathered from several research papers clearly indicated that this made each isometric exercise more effective while at the same time minimising overall negative stress.

The maximum 10 second rest period is just enough to allow the muscle being exercised to almost recover before the next exercise is applied. Naturally, this will place a high demand on the cardiovascular system of anyone performing this system. If this is an issue, either increase the rest time and/or reduce the level of applied intensity during each isometric exercise accordingly. The objective would then be to gradually improve by decreasing the rest time between exercises while increasing the level of intensity that is applied. Eventually, your overall fitness level will increase to allow you to perform higher intensity exercises during each phase of the TRISOmetric™ exercise set you are performing.

Never be tempted to perform more sets because this can be counterproductive. If you feel the need to do more, then it is always better to apply even greater intensity to each isometric exercise while decreasing the speed of the already super-slow portion even more. As a general guide, if you feel that you can perform another set of the TRISOmetric™ exercise, then you have not been performing it correctly. Remember, intensity and force are both inversely proportional. As the level of exercise intensity and/or force increases during an exercise, then the length of time that exercise can be performed will proportionally decrease.

Initially, we also recommend that you perform only basic exercises for each body part. For example, you can perform either a power rack squat, wall squat, or an Iso-Bow® squat in 3 positions as isometric exercises. One position could be while your thighs are parallel to the floor, the next position about 20 degrees higher, and the last position about 20 degrees higher again. With those completed, you could then perform a Bullworker® squat, a power rack bar squat, or simply a freehand squat – all in super-slow exercise style.

Another example would be to perform a combination of an Iso-Bow®, Bullworker® or Steel Bow® chest press as an isometric exercise in three positions over the calculated range of motion. Then, after these have been completed, aim to perform 10 isotonic repetitions in super-slow exercise style using either the Bullworker®, the Steel Bow or by performing push-ups from either the toes or the knees. Once you have mastered achieving the 3 equal isometric exercise positions for each TRISOmetric™ exercise, then you have quite a wide selection of isotonic exercises to choose from to complete the exercise. Please note: TRISOmetric™ exercise program calls for 10 isotonic repetitions in super-slow motion, with my Muscle Up for Menopause program, I suggest three repetitions.

Super-Slow Training

I believe that it is almost impossible to move too slowly during an isotonic resistance exercise, however, it is easily possible to move too quickly. Super-slow is a form of strength training that was made popular by Ken Hutchins who worked at Nautilus and is based on an original concept by Dr Vincent Bocchicchio.

Dr Bocchicchio proposed that a single repetition of resistance training should take 10 seconds for the lifting phase, which is the concentric contraction where the muscles shorten. Then, pausing slightly to prevent momentum from being generated, after which it would take another 10 seconds to complete the lowering, or eccentric phase, where the muscles lengthen.

The super-slow concept incorporates extremely slow repetition speeds when compared to traditional resistance training protocols. In super-slow training, the emphasis is on minimizing momentum through minimal acceleration which, in turn, improves muscular loading. Most research suggests that super-slow training yields much better results in terms of strength gains and muscle growth than traditional resistance training methods.

The heart of the super-slow concept is based on the amount of tension a muscle develops. This is directly affected by the speed at which the muscle lengthens during the eccentric or lowering phase or shortens during the concentric or lifting phase of an exercise. The more tension that is generated, the more muscle fibres that are recruited. More importantly, the slower the myosin and actin filaments within the muscle fibres slide past each other, the more links that are formed between the filaments. Using super-slow exercise speeds a maximum amount of tension is generated and a higher number of filament links are formed. In short, super-slow training activates more muscle fibres at an increased rate to maintain the force necessary to move the resistance provided. This is why it is a very efficient way to increase both strength and muscle size.

A typical super-slow workout would consist of one set of each exercise which is performed to the point of complete muscle fatigue/failure. A 10-repetition exercise in such a routine would take around 200 to 250 seconds to perform in practice, with the overall workout session taking no longer than 30 minutes to complete. Since this is a high-intensity system, it requires greater rest time between workout sessions. Therefore, a workout frequency of twice each week is typically recommended to avoid overtraining and burnout.

One of the great advantages of super-slow training is in injury prevention. This is because in traditional resistance training, to make it more challenging more weight is added to increase the resistance used. Therefore, in and of itself, the traditional method naturally increases the risk of injury.

With super-slow training, to make the exercise more challenging and engage more muscle fibres, simply slow the exercise down even more without there being a need to increase the weight.

A by-product of super-slow training is that it also produces some excellent cardiovascular benefits. This is because the heart is an involuntary muscle, it will always pump harder when there is more blood that needs pumping. Several studies have shown that super-slow training returns more blood to the heart than traditional aerobic training methods.

Strength at Only One Angle?

I have written quite a lot about dividing the ROM or Range of Motion of a limb roughly equally into three positions and then performing an isometric exercise at each point. I thought I would make this clearer in pictures. Also, to explain away a common myth that isometric contraction exercises will only increase muscle strength at the specific angle at which the muscle and joint are exercised. When talking about building strength in a broader range, rather than at a more specific point, one of the first things that should also be remembered is that during regular isotonic weight training, a constant-curve range of strength gain is not achieved anyway. The data clearly shows that in respect of isometric exercise, it is only partially true that there is only an increase in strength at the angle the contraction is engaged. The scientific study performed by scientists Kitai and Sale called: "Specificity of Joint Angle in Isometric Training," concluded that strength gains were the greatest at the specific angle the training was performed. It also concluded that there was a significant increase in strength along a much wider strength curve than previously thought. The study showed that there were increases in strength at the angles of +5 degrees, and -5 degrees to the isometric hold position.

More extensive studies have subsequently found that with isometric contraction exercises there is often an even wider strength curve benefit than was first thought. The later studies found that between 20% and 50% of strength transfer occurs at the angles of +20 degrees, and -20 degrees to the isometric hold position. This is huge, and it completely dispels all myths about any potential issues about this. The additional research also concluded that for those athletes who wanted to achieve the most complete and constant curve strength gain, it was comparatively easy to achieve with isometric contraction exercises, especially when compared to regular isotonic weight training. In practical terms, to achieve the most complete and constant-curve strength gain possible, an advanced athlete would simply perform an isometric contraction exercise at two, three, or many more positions along the ROM of the body part being exercised. A normal, healthy limb has a certain Range of Motion, AKA: ROM. This is the arc through which the movement takes place at a joint, or series of joints. This ROM is technically called "Osteokinematic" motion. Taking the biceps curl as an example, the range of motion for that movement in the pictures starts at zero when the hand is in the lower position and goes up to approximately 130 degrees in the upper position.

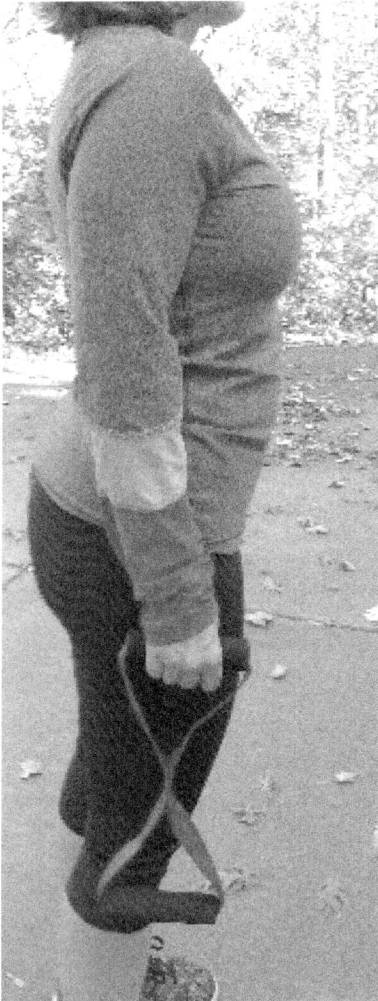 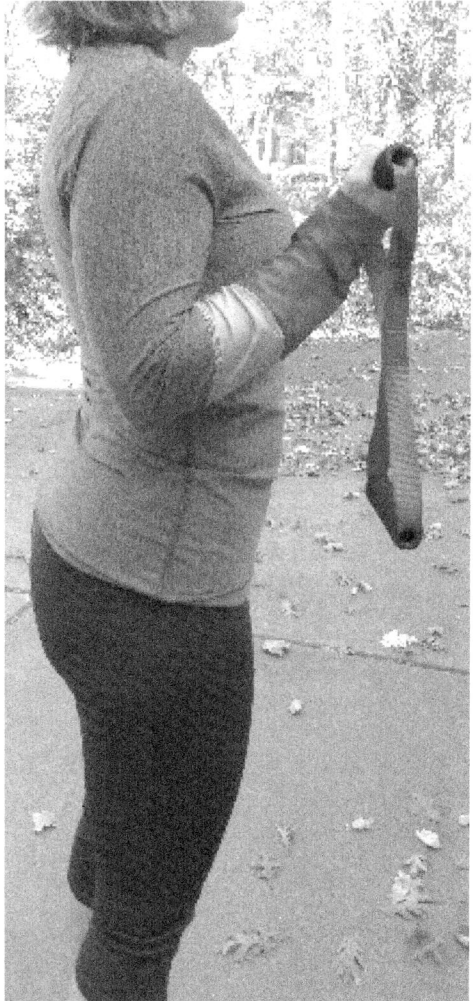

| Zero Degrees | 130 Degrees |

Assuming that there is a strength-curve benefit of +20 degrees and -20 degrees around the point at which an isometric contraction is performed, then the first position would be at approximately 20 degrees from the neutral starting point because this would give a strength-curve benefit covering the first 40 degrees of the ROM.

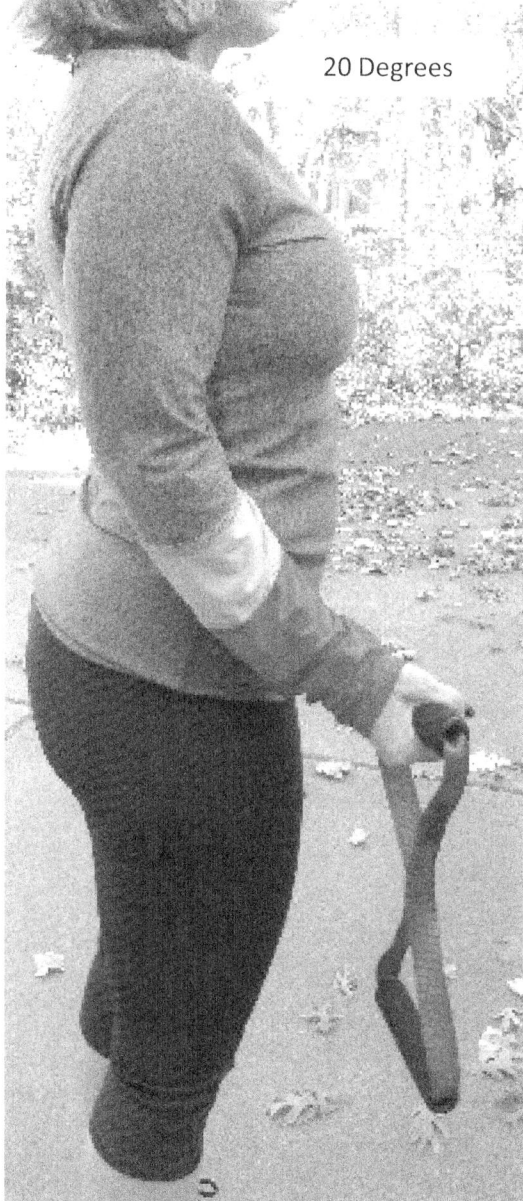

20 Degrees

The second position would be at approximately 50 degrees from the starting point which would safely overlap the first strength-curve arc from about the 30-degree point and extend up to about 70 degrees.

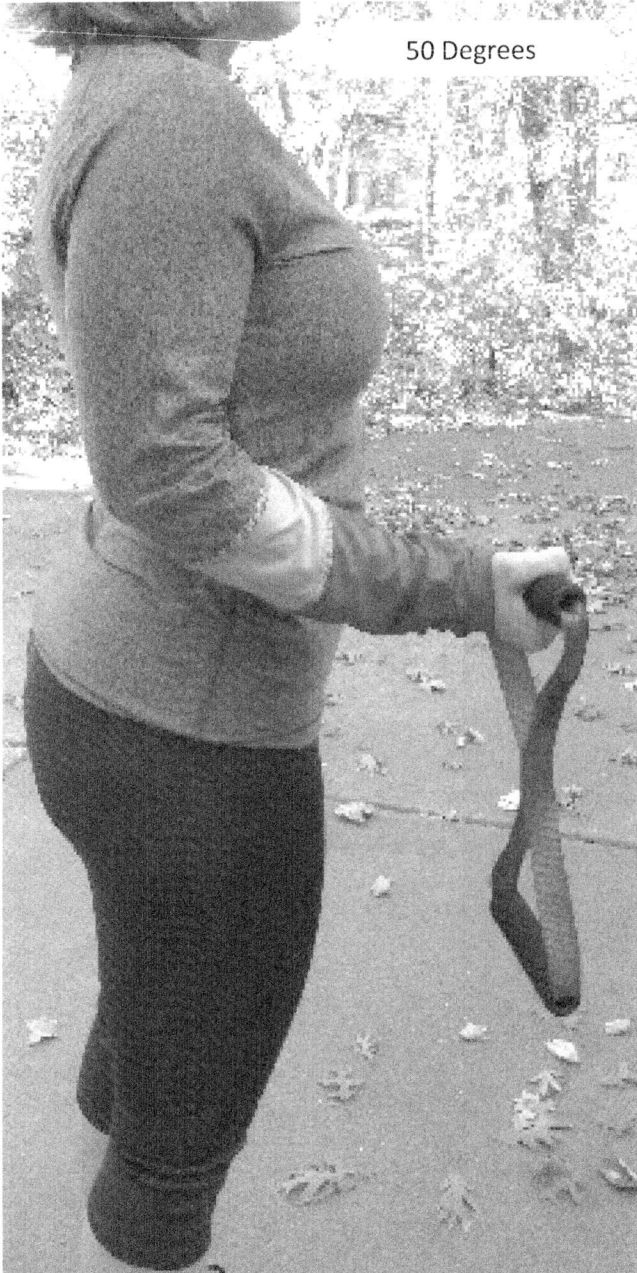

50 Degrees

The final position is at approximately 80 to 95 degrees from the starting point, overlapping the last point to provide a strength-curve benefit at the high end of the arc at circa 130-degree of the maximum ROM.

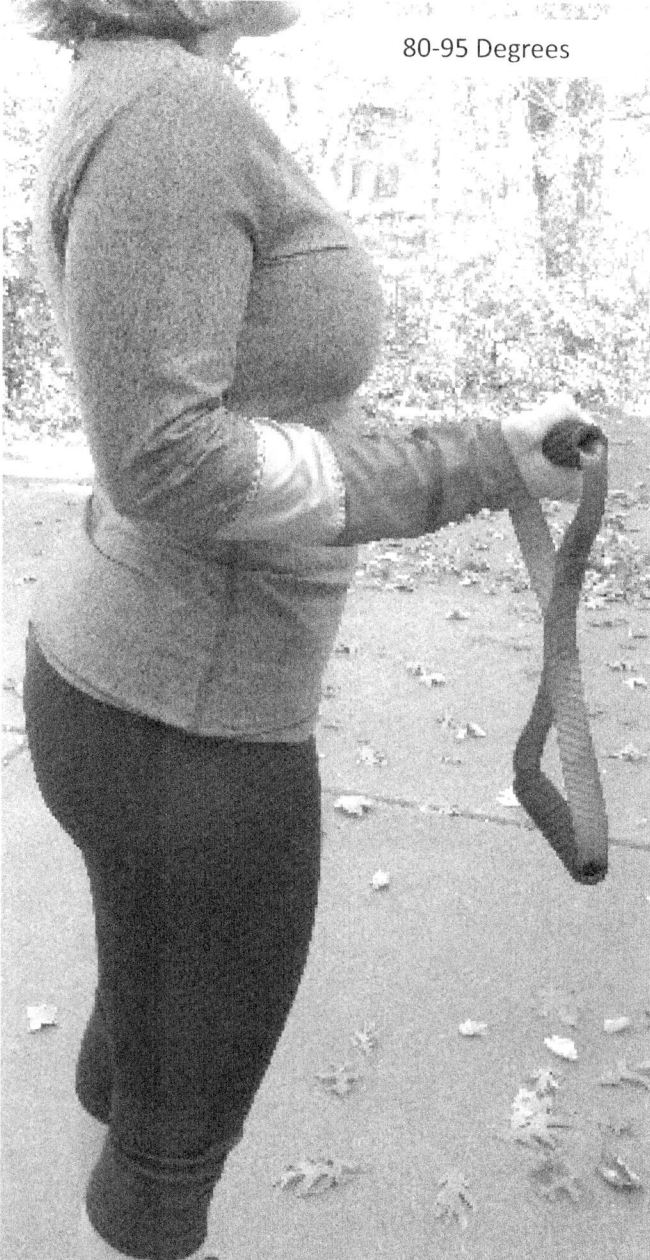

80-95 Degrees

If necessary, a highly advanced athlete might also want to add an isometric contraction exercise at both the starting and end position of the ROM. This would then strengthen the muscles when in the most mechanically disadvantaged position.

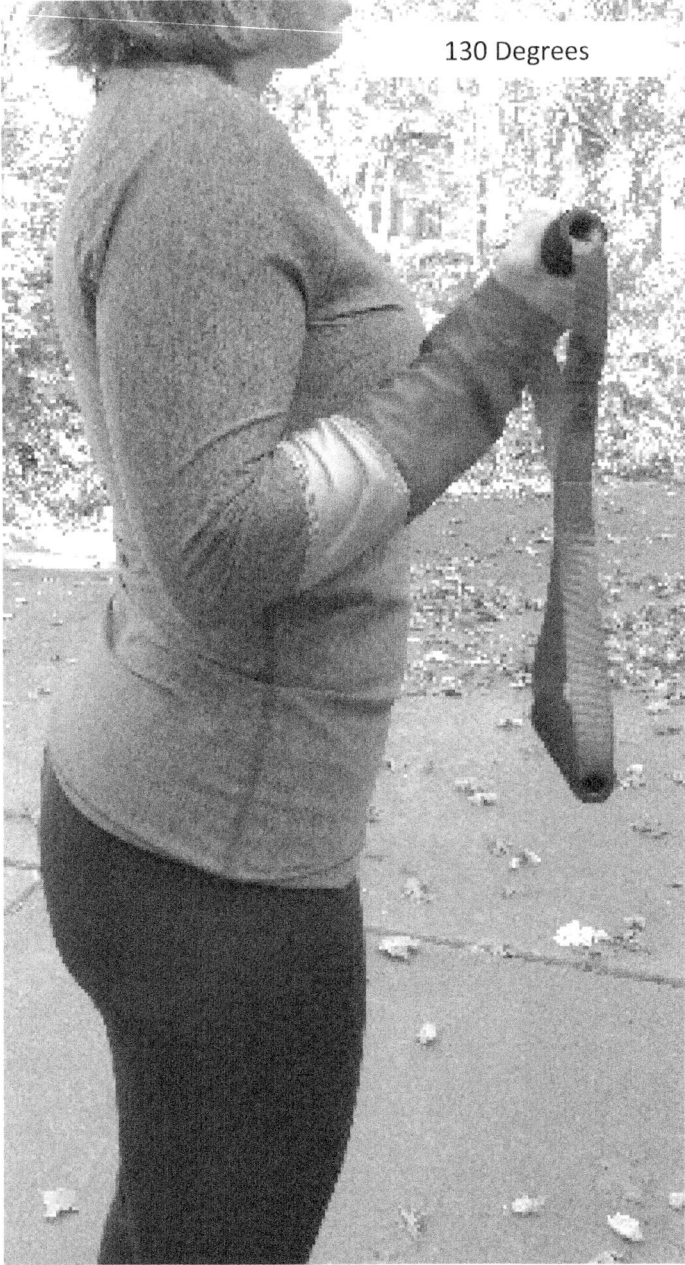

130 Degrees

Chapter 4. All Things Iso-Bow®

A common question we are asked is: "is it necessary to use the Iso-Bow® to perform an effective isometric or self-resisted workout?" This is a good question. No, it is not necessary to use an Iso-Bow®, but we believe that it is better if you do, and there are several reasons why.

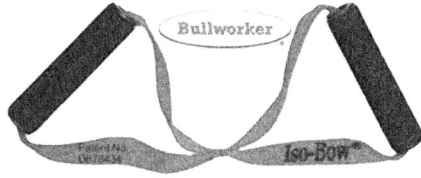

Firstly, it is all about the science and safety of biomechanics. A stable line of biomechanical progression all begins with a correctly positioned grip, a firm grip, and the progression in continuing that stability through correctly aligned joints and limbs while you perform the exercise. The same is true in isometric exercise because it all begins with a stable line of biomechanical progression. This starts with either a properly clenched hand or fist and continuing that stability through correctly aligned joints and limbs to perform the isometric hold.

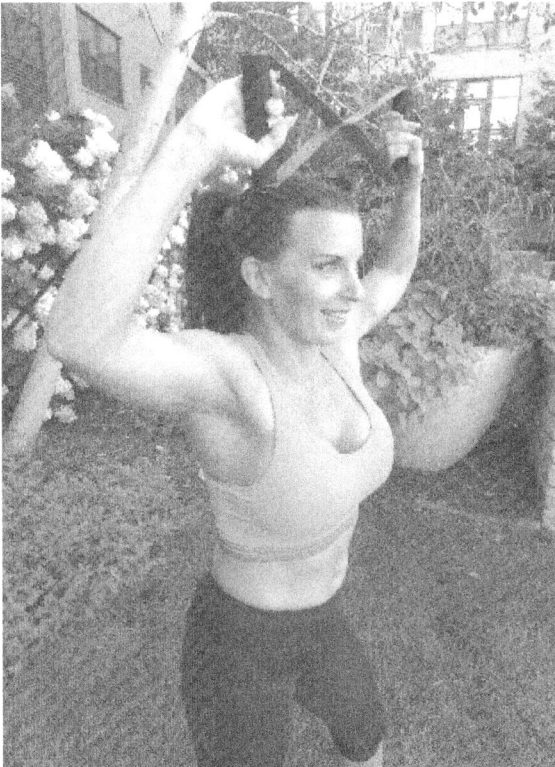

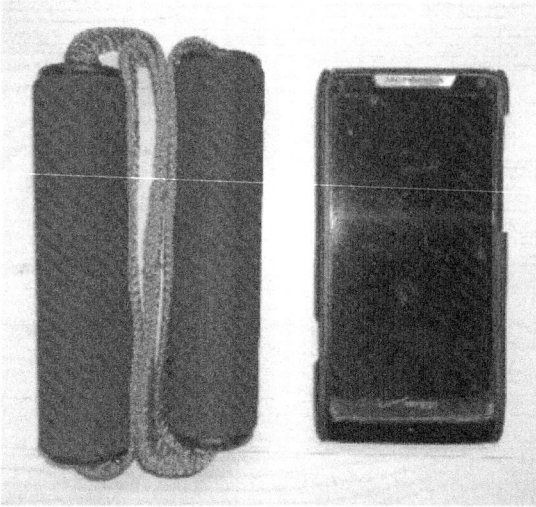

This is just one reason why we fully recommend and endorse the Iso-Bow® because it makes this entire process much easier. It has a well-designed and comfortable non-slip handgrip, which allows you to execute a firm, stable handgrip position to begin creating a stable line of biomechanical progression.

The Iso-Bow® is a product we fully endorse and highly recommend. It is inexpensive, high quality, and it works exceptionally well. An amazing Iso-Bow® costs "pennies" in comparison to other exercise devices, and even a pair of them can easily fit into your pocket, they never need adjusting, they can deliver a total-body workout at the perfect level of intensity for either a complete unfit beginner or an advanced athlete!

If you have already read "The 70 Second Difference™" book, then

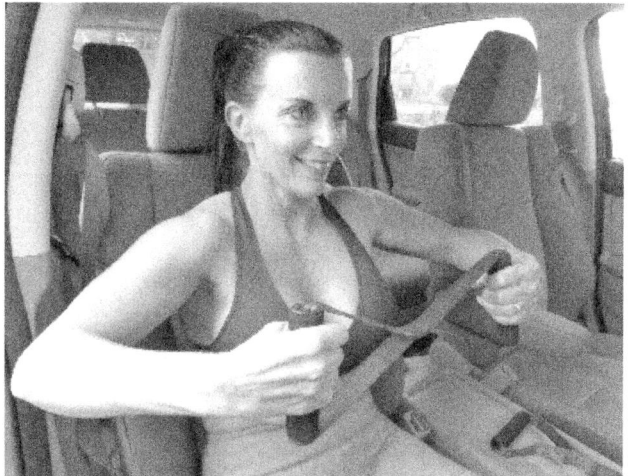

you will also know that we are not even endorsing our product. We are simply endorsing a product which we believe will be the best investment you will ever make if you want to get fit, strong, and in the best shape of your life. The company that makes the Iso-Bow® is Hughes Marketing LLC, and they also produce a small range of other highly effective exercise products, which all deliver excellent results at a fair price.

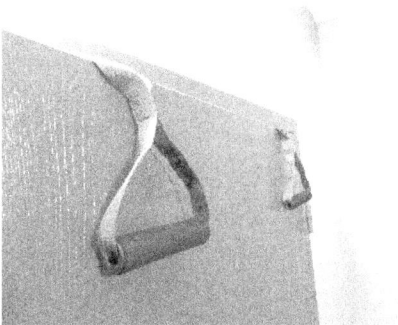

The Iso-Bow® is versatile too, and it can be used with equal effectiveness as both an isotonic, and an isometric exercise device. It allows the user to perform highly effective self-resisted isotonic exercises for almost every muscle group.

A pair of Iso-Bows® can even be used as a great doorway pull-up device, which can even fold up and

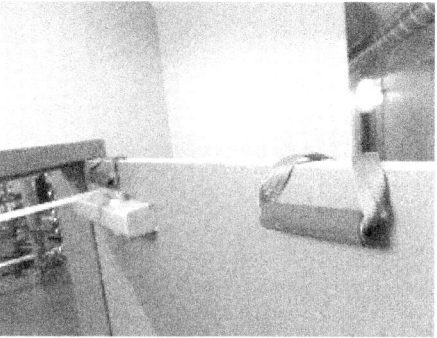

slip right into your pocket when you are done. Try doing that with a regular, clumsy steel doorway pull-up bar!

The Iso-Bow® is naturally a first-class isometric exercise device, and it allows a very wide range of exercises to be performed that work almost every muscle group of the body. It also allows the effective execution of more advanced techniques to be performed within the isometric exercise system.

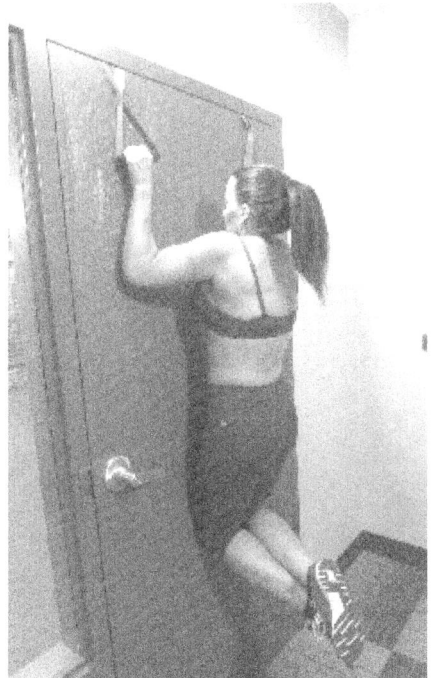

Since the Iso-Bow® is inexpensive, well designed, well-constructed, and extremely useful in ways we have not even begun to describe here in this book, it is not so much a recommendation for you to get a pair, rather an instruction for you to do so. We believe that you will soon see why these inexpensive devices are what we believe to be the finest, most versatile, and most powerful of all exercise devices that have ever been invented!

That is a bold statement, but it is made because of our sincere belief in the product, and how you will benefit from owning a pair if you use them correctly. Do not forget, we do not make this product, we simply believe in it with that degree of commitment.

Securing the Iso-Bow® With Your Feet

When performing leg exercises such as squats and lunges, as well as lower back and glute exercises such as the deadlift, it becomes necessary to properly secure the Iso-Bow® using your feet.

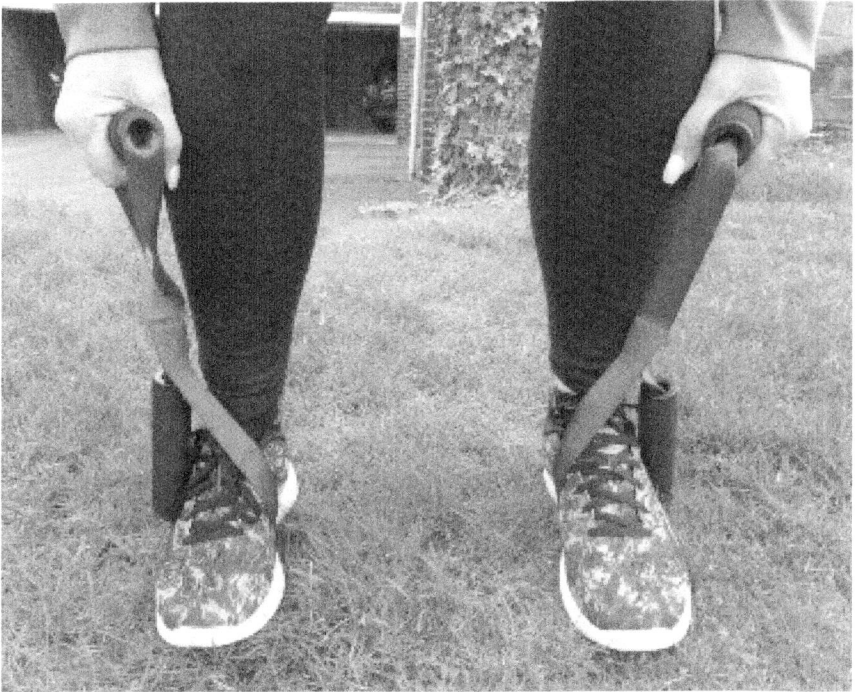

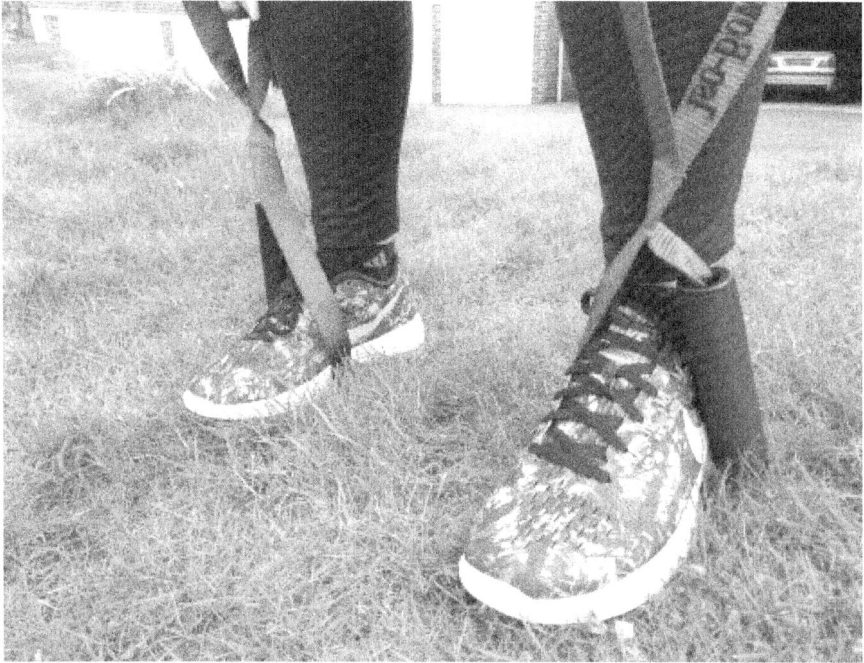

There are several ways in which the Iso-Bow® can be secured using your feet, and your personal preference of how you do this will depend upon many factors such as your foot size, your choice of footwear, and ease of operation. You can secure the Iso-Bow® with your foot inside one of the handles. You do this by adjusting the handgrip to one side, usually the outer side of the foot, and then place your feet inside the loop like a stirrup.

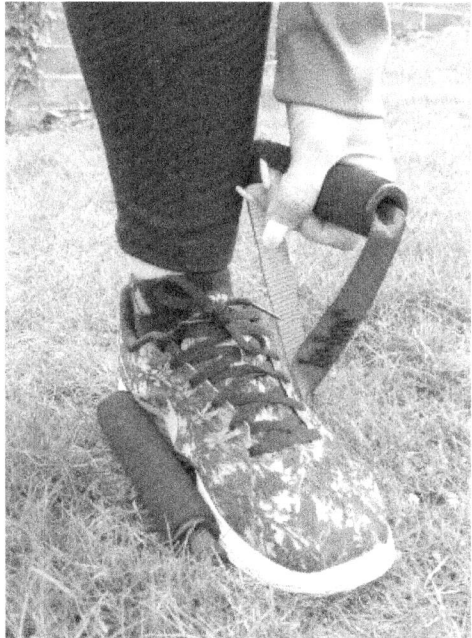

Another method is to place the Iso-Bow® flat on the

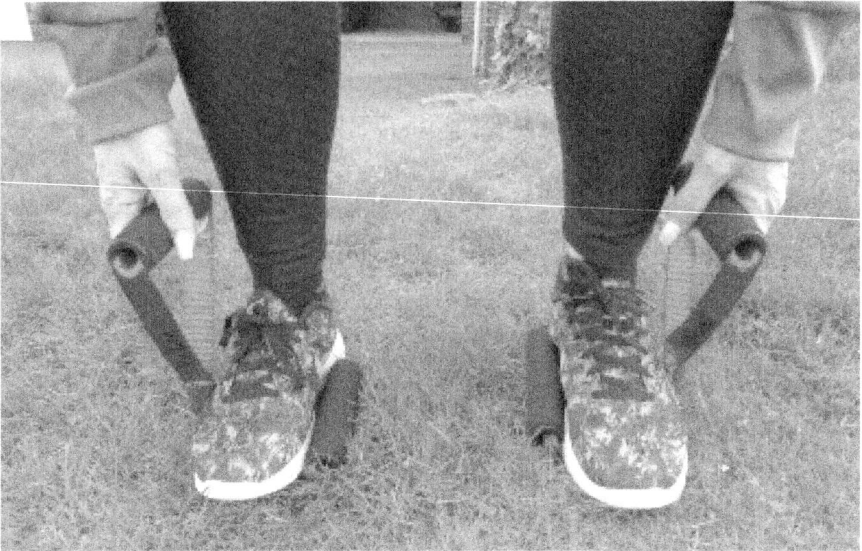

floor and then stand on one side of the straps so that the handle of the same side sits flush to your inner foot. In this position, it will be your bodyweight combined with the handle pressing against the inner side of your foot which enables you to pull safely and securely.

The final method is to simply place each foot through one end of an Iso-Bow®, stepping onto the foam handgrip as you do so. This method is slightly less stable than the other two methods. However, if the foot can be pushed far enough through the loop of the Iso-Bow® handle, then the handle will slightly

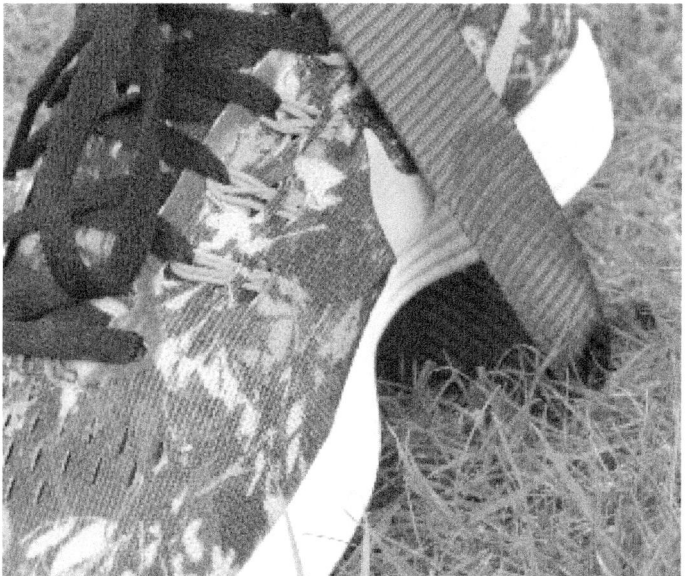

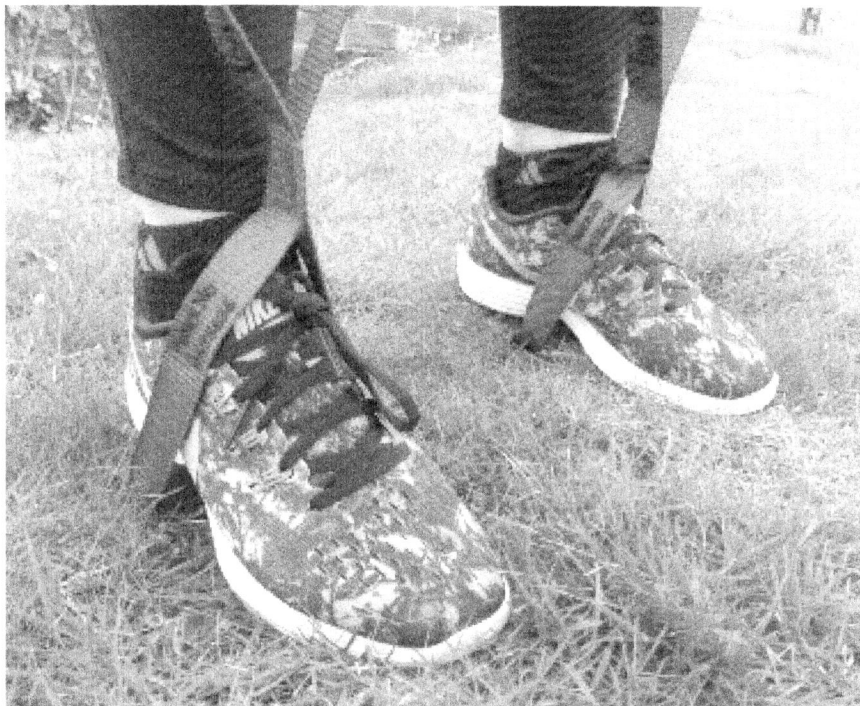

raise the level of your heel making it easier for some people to squat or lunge. Naturally, safety is always a top priority so whichever method you ultimately choose to use, you should always make sure that when securing the Iso-Bow® with your feet that there is never any chance of it slipping in any way while you exercise.

Shortening The Iso-Bow® - The Cradle

Generally, the Iso-Bow® is the ideal size for most people to use with each exercise. However, occasionally you may prefer to reduce its operational size by roughly half, by creating what we call an Iso-Bow® cradle.

To do this you place one of the handles inside the webbing loop of the other handle side of the device. The handle you have just placed inside the loop is then cradled by the webbing and can be gripped as normal. Your thumb, and fingers can then wrap around both the foam handle and the webbing of the cradle loop to help ensure an even firmer grip position is created.

This reduced size allows for an even greater operational range within the movement capability of each limb/joint to be created for certain exercises. These include The Cross-Chest Press, the Upper Back Power Pull, and the Biceps and Triceps Cradle Press-Curl.

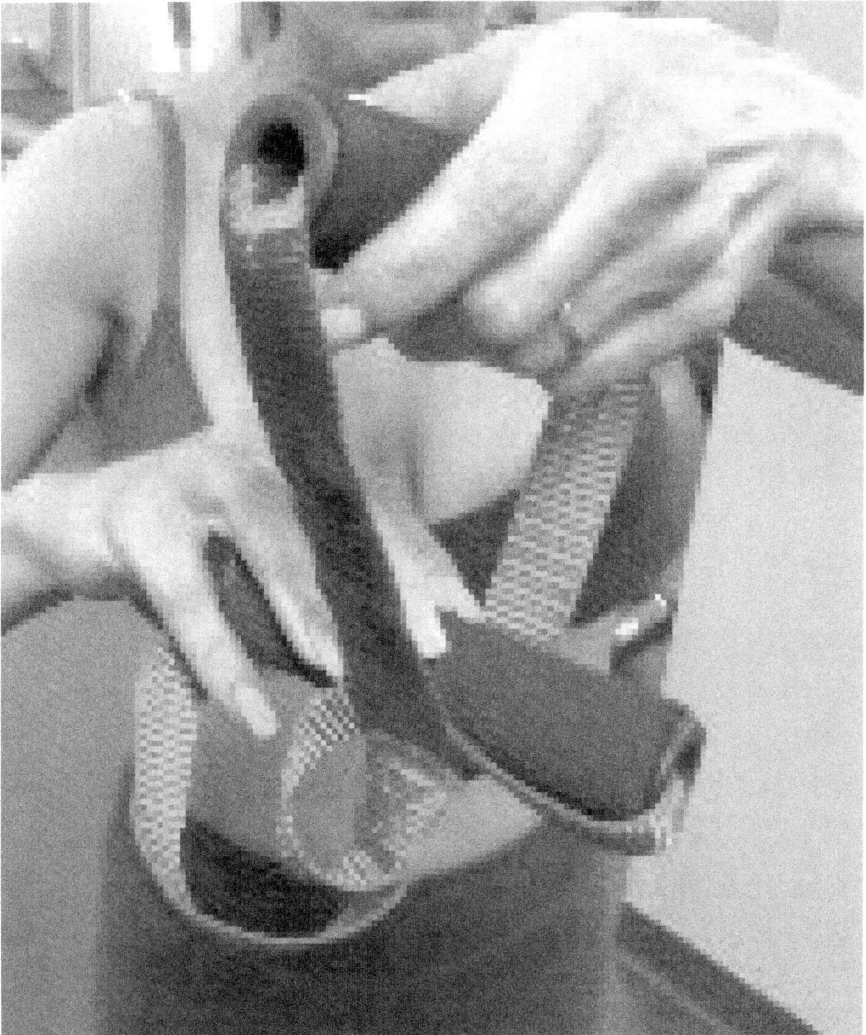

Proprietary and Readily Available Equipment

The Bullworker® Classic

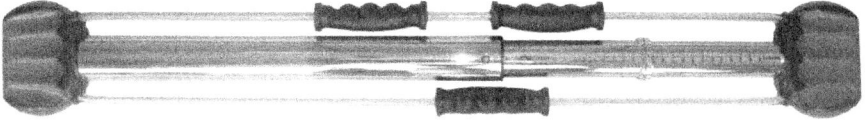

The Bullworker® Classic is approximately 36 inches long and can be used either as a stand-alone device or as a complete home gym when in combination with the Steel Bow® and the Iso-Bow®. It currently has several interchangeable springs with different levels of resistance. These may be added to in the future to allow an even greater range of people to use the device for an even wider range of exercises. Today, with the shift towards more people choosing to exercise at home, the Bullworker has now become the total-body all-in-one compact personal gym of choice.

The Steel Bow®

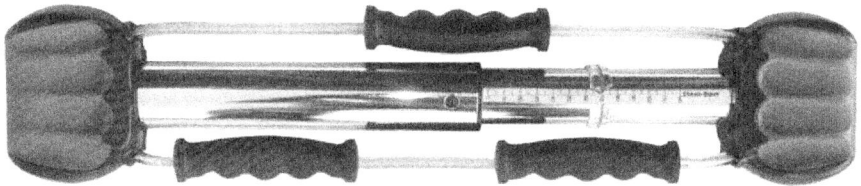

The Steel Bow® is about 20 inches long and is simply a shorter version for the full-size Bullworker® Classic model. The Steel Bow® comes with several interchangeable springs of varying levels of resistance.

IIEDs or Improvised Isometric Exercise Devices

One of the best things about isometric exercises is that if you do not want to use traditional gym equipment or proprietary devices, then you do not have to use them to perform a full workout. Instead, you can either use nothing at all except your own body, immovable objects such as doors, walls, and door jambs, or readily available everyday items.

These can include walking sticks/poles, broom handles, towels and sturdy towing, or a climbing rope. I will outline some of these items as suggestions for alternative equipment/devices you can use for your workout sessions.

The Walking Stick/Pole

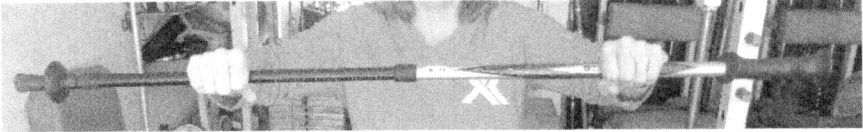

The walking stick or pro-style walking pole is an excellent device to use for an isometric workout. It is basically the equivalent of a barbell or Bullworker® Classic without the steel cables at each side. One of the great advantages the pro-style walking pole offers is that it can be adjusted to various lengths, which make it easily adaptable for use in a variety of exercises. Many of the exercises can be performed alone, without any need for partner assistance. An even greater range of exercises can be performed if a workout partner is available. Nordic Walking Poles are slightly different from ordinary walking poles, but they work equally well for isometric exercises.

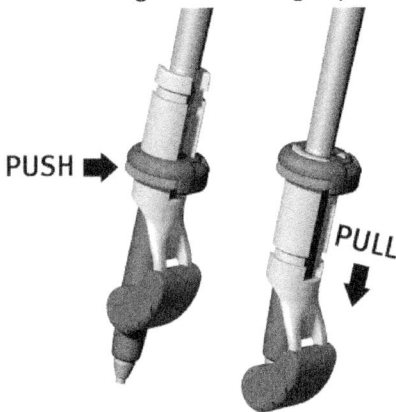

PUSH ➡

PULL

Nordic Walking Pole Tip by: Tslmarketing

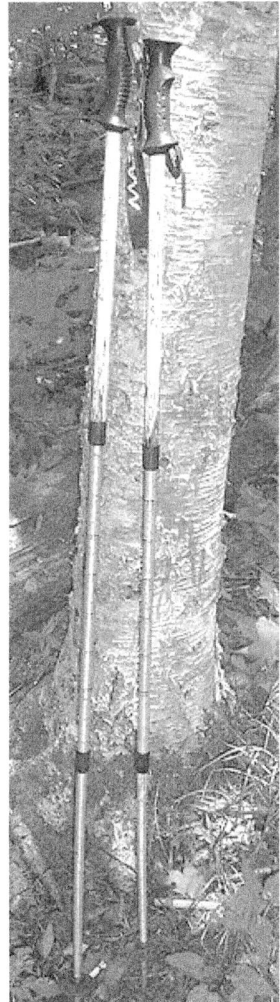

Photo: Daniel Case

The Humble Beach or Bath Towel

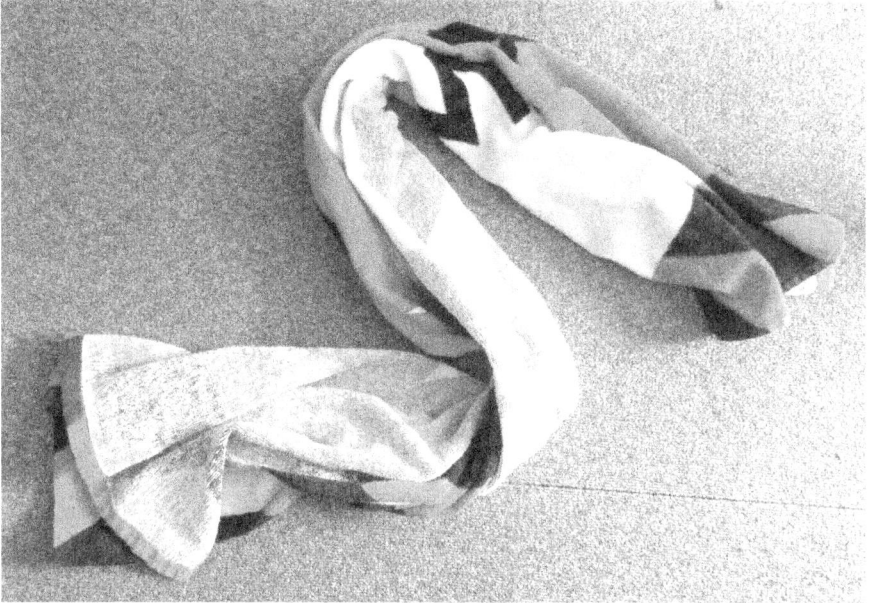

The humble beach or bath towel is a common tool used by isometric enthusiasts who have nothing else to exercise with. It is also an exercise tool of choice for many because it is incredibly versatile.

When choosing a towel to exercise with, the important things to look for are that it must be long enough, it must also be flexible enough to enable you to grip it properly, therefore, it must not be too thick. Naturally, it must also be in good condition and not be liable to tear or rip during your exercise session.

Rope – Either Climbing Rope or Towing Rope

A rope is another remarkably simple but highly effective tool that can be used to perform an isometric and/or self-resisted workout routine. the important things to look for in a rope that might be suitable for exercise use are, sufficient length, it must be thick enough to allow a comfortable handgrip, and it must be in good condition so that it will not break during your workout routine.

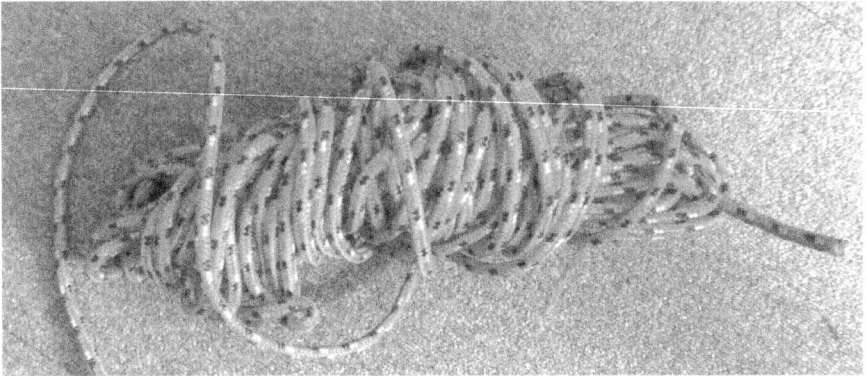

If you are using your feet to secure the rope, then for added safety and comfort you may wish to loop the rope around the foot as shown. This will make it less likely to slip when it is pulled hard, and it will be more comfortable for the foot as well.

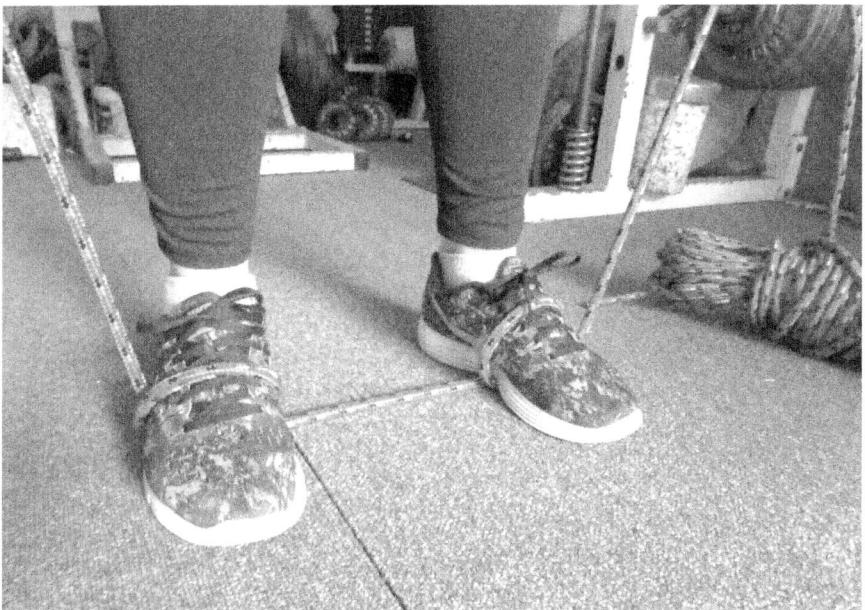

The Broom Handle

The broom handle can be used almost identically to the walking stick or pro-style walking pole. By its very nature, it is not nearly as flexible as a walking stick or pro-style walking pole.

This is because since you can easily take a walking stick or pro-style walking pole virtually anywhere because that is precisely what they have been designed for.

You would appear to be very odd indeed if you were to carry around a broom with you to exercise with, whereas a walking stick or pro-style walking pole would not look even the slighted bit out of place.

If you use a broom handle at home to exercise with, then make sure it is solid and will not break when used in a workout routine.

Also, we would strongly caution against using one to support your body weight in any way with the broom handle to support it.

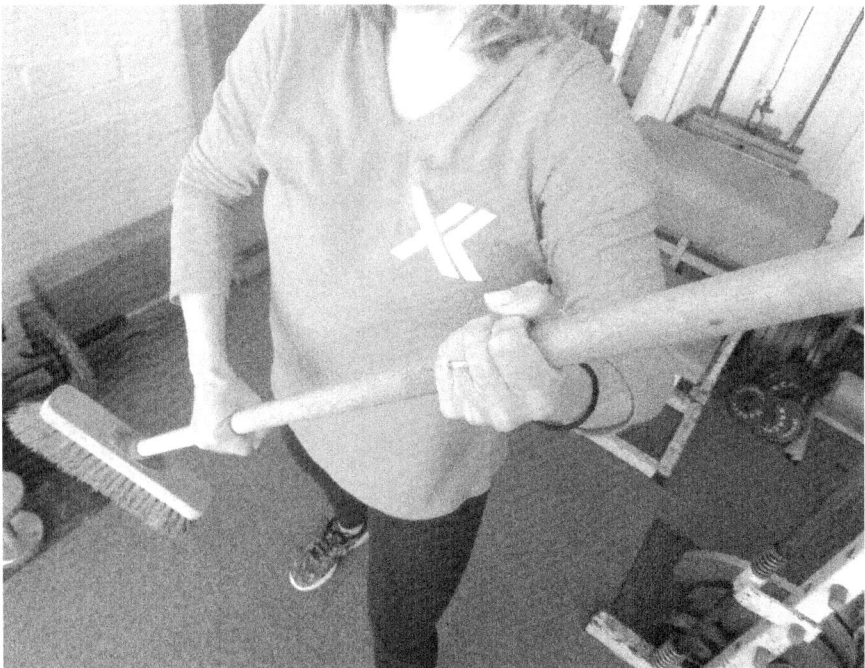

The Climber's Sling

The climber's sling, or any kind of climbing grade webbing/material for that matter, almost always makes an ideal IIED or Improvised Isometric Exercise Device. A climbing sling, or runner, is an item of basic equipment climbers use. It is either a tied or sewn loop of webbing that can be attached to a carabiner or around a rock and hitched (tied) to other equipment. Climber's slings are extremely useful because the longer ones can be easily double-looped, or more, to reduce their circumference by half with every reducing loop added. This makes the longer slings an extremely versatile IIED because the length and thickness can be so easily and quickly adjusted according to the isometric exercise you wish to perform.

Professionally sewn and bonded climber's slings are extremely strong with a typical average breaking strength of at least 22 kilonewtons or 4,900 lbf. To give you a better frame of reference to the breaking strain of a 22 kN climbing sling, an average Range Rover Sport SUV weighs about 4,727 lb or 2,144 kg. Therefore, a typical 22 kN climbing sling made from nylon webbing is more than capable of being used safely as an IIED, or any other kind of exercise for that matter. When undamaged and properly made, they cannot be ripped apart during exercise, or by any other form of human muscle power, not even by The World's Strongest Man.

The Climber's Daisy Chain

Another excellent and versatile IIED or Improvised Isometric Exercise Device found in the typical range of equipment sold in a climbing store is the daisy chain.

A daisy chain is a webbing chain strap that is several feet/centimetres long. Typically, it is made from

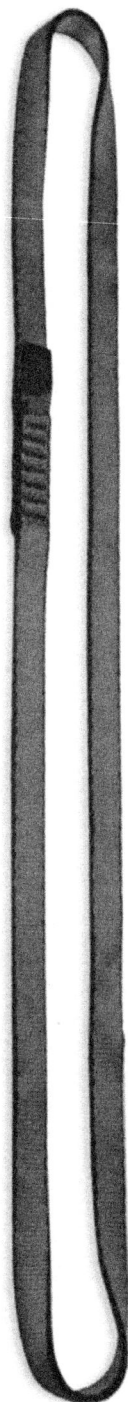

approximately one-inch (2.54 cm) nylon webbing of the same or similar type to that used in climbing slings and lengthening straps between anchor points and the main climbing rope.

The webbing is securely stitched at intervals of approximately two inches to form loops on one side along the length of the main webbing strap.

Alternatively, and these are the type we prefer, the nylon webbing is sewn into a series of closely spaced interlocked loops to create a looped daisy chain for the desired length of the device.

At one end there is usually a much larger foot loop to accommodate a climbing boot, and at the other end, there is a carabiner point made from a smaller piece of nylon webbing in a tight loop or bite.

A Typical Climber's Daisy Chain

Note the Foot Loop at One End and the Carabiner Point/s at the Other End

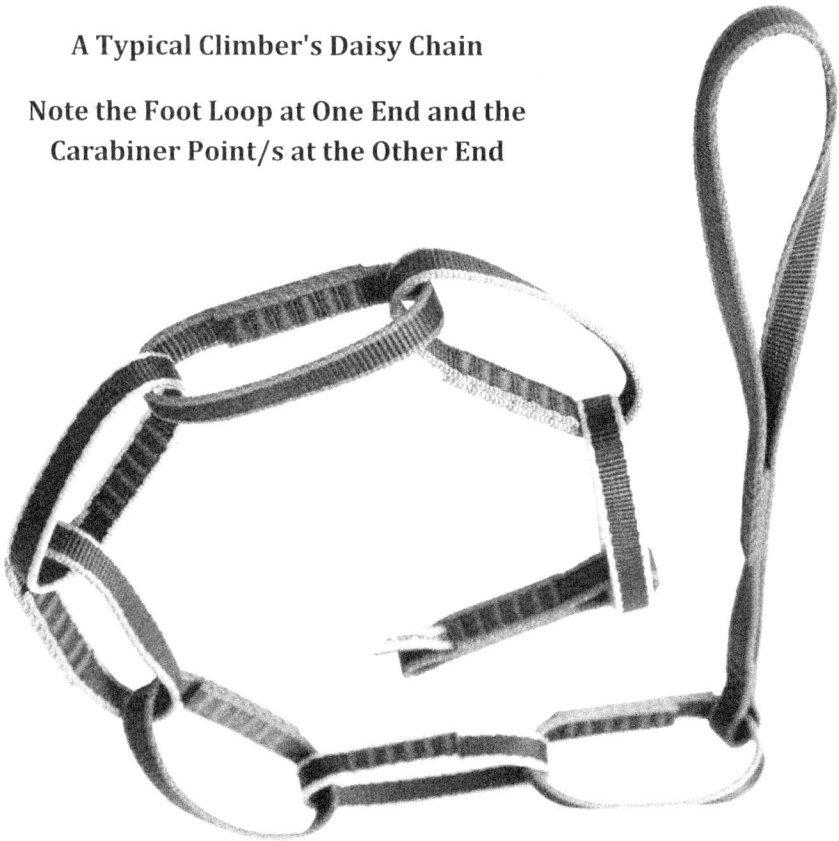

Section Conclusion

Since the isometric exercise requires no limb movement, it is extremely easy to perform a wide range of effective exercises using the self-resistance method.

Therefore, one can use just about any device that is unbreakable by human muscle power alone. However, as with all things, using a proprietary device that is purpose-made will always make it easier, and sometimes safer to perform.

One of the good things about all of the example devices shown in this section is that none could be considered to be expensive, and all are built to a high standard of quality and durability. In short, the choice is yours and whatever you choose will deliver good results!

Chapter 5.

Things to Remember and Tips Before You Begin

- The first and perhaps the most important thing to remember is: **NEVER HOLD YOUR BREATH AT ANY TIME.**
- Breathing in and out naturally during all isometric exercises will also help you count the number of elapsed seconds much more accurately, with one full breath in and out taking approximately one second.
- We recommend that you read the instructions about each exercise carefully. You can also watch the associated videos via the TWiEA™ website if you wish to become a member and access those resources.
- Always leave a safe distance between you and others if exercising with any proprietary device or IIED (Improvised Isometric Exercise Device)
- Always check the structural integrity of any type of exercise device. If there is any doubt about the structural integrity, then do not use it for exercise or any other purpose.
- Double-check that any/all adjustable joints on the exercise device and/or IIED are secure before use.
- Weight loss/fat loss will ONLY occur when any exercise plan is used in conjunction with a calorie-controlled diet.
- It is critically important to completely focus your mind on the exercise being performed. Envision the muscle you are exercising is growing larger and stronger.
- Always consult a professional coach to devise a detailed stretching routine, this will ensure that you are stretching the areas effectively rather than risking injury.
- Always ensure that a stable line of biomechanical progression is achieved before engaging in and performing any exercise.

△ Warming-up, stretching, and cooling down are three of the most overlooked yet essential elements to exercise, and we cannot stress their importance strongly enough.

△ During ANY form of physical exercise, including isometrics, if you apply too much intensity too soon, then you may inadvertently strain a muscle. Isometric exercise can be intense, and a single isometric exercise engages a great many more muscle fibres than even high-intensity weight training does, and at a much higher level too.

For safety's sake, we recommend using Dynamic Flexation™ to engage your muscles gradually and progressively into ANY exercise according to our ISOfitness Exercise Engagement Timeline™.

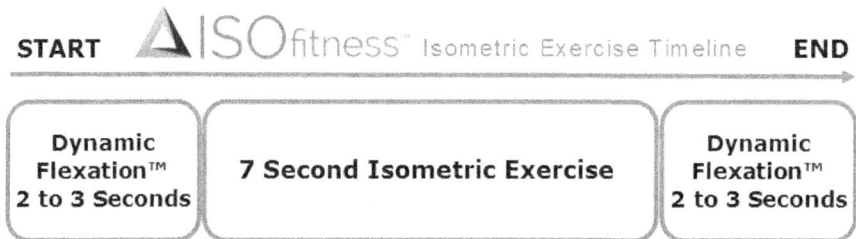

START △ISOfitness™ Isometric Exercise Timeline **END**

Dynamic Flexation™ 2 to 3 Seconds	7 Second Isometric Exercise	Dynamic Flexation™ 2 to 3 Seconds

The main benefit of properly warming-up for several minutes before a workout is injury prevention and increasing your heart rate and circulation to your muscles, ligaments, and tendons. In addition to properly warming-up, always perform a gentle flex and stretch of the muscles and joints which are about to be exercised. For example, squatting down fully to flex the thighs and loosen the knees is always a good idea before performing any leg exercises.

Dynamic Flexation™ performed before any exercise should help to ensure greater great flexibility and increased blood supply to the muscles and surrounding tissue. It is important to remember that warming-up and stretching are two different concepts and that stretching is not a good warm-up. This is because stretching will put the muscle in an uncontracted position and weaken it. Stretching is always best performed after a workout has been completed, together with a proper cool-down regimen.

Charts of the Major Muscle Groups

The following charts showing the major muscle groups should help you to better identify the ones you are targeting in each exercise. The better acquainted you become with the muscle groups and their basic function, then the better your exercise style should become.

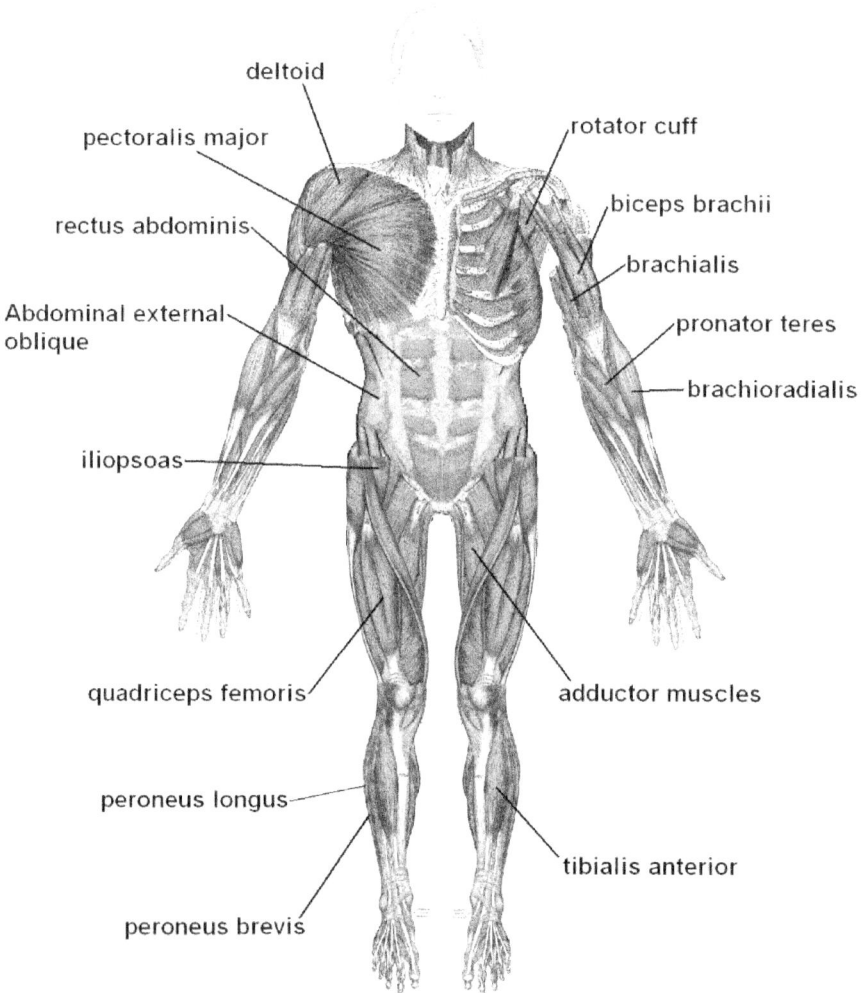

deltoid

pectoralis major

rotator cuff

biceps brachii

rectus abdominis

brachialis

Abdominal external oblique

pronator teres

brachioradialis

iliopsoas

quadriceps femoris

adductor muscles

peroneus longus

tibialis anterior

peroneus brevis

Frontal (anterior) View of the Main Human Skeletal Muscles

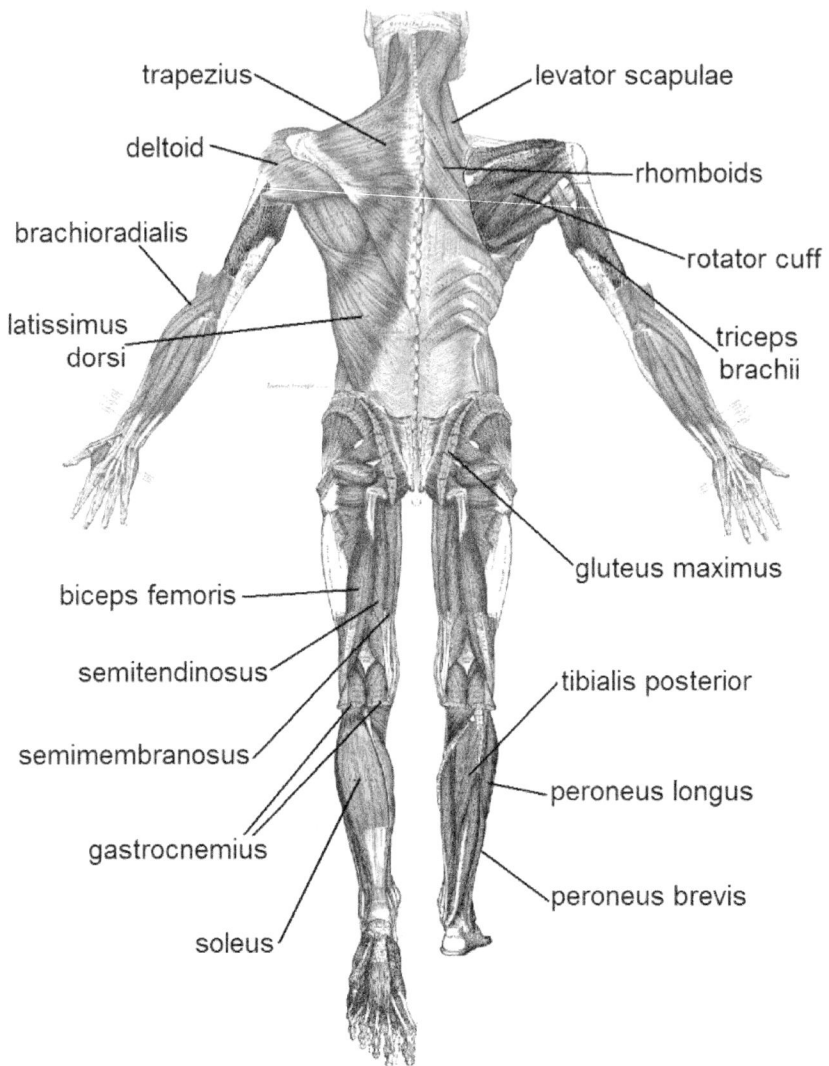

Rear (posterior) View of the Main Human Skeletal Muscles

Labels: trapezius, levator scapulae, deltoid, rhomboids, brachioradialis, rotator cuff, latissimus dorsi, triceps brachii, gluteus maximus, biceps femoris, semitendinosus, tibialis posterior, semimembranosus, peroneus longus, gastrocnemius, peroneus brevis, soleus

Isometric exercises are deceptively powerful. Even when engaging in what may feel like only moderate-intensity exercise, you are probably still engaging and contracting many more muscle fibres than you would in a similar isotonic exercise. If you are in any doubt whatsoever, then always perform the exercise with a little less intensity.

All exercises and workout plans work equally well for men and women. Both sexes can build strength, muscle, body build, or simply get into great shape if so desired, each according to their natural ability.

In our resource books, the exercises listed are suggestions of what can be performed for each body part/muscle group. We are not suggesting that they should all be performed. Instead, users may wish to select the most suitable exercises from each section. In our course books, please perform the exercises according to the workout session notes.

Finally, please read, review, and ensure that you have fully complied with all recommendations in the section headed, Important General Safety and Health Guidelines.

Finally, only start using the isometric, or any other exercise system with the full approval of your physician.

Chapter 6. About the Exercise Model

Unless you have skipped the entire first part of this book, you will already know a great deal about me. For those who have skipped that section to get right down to the exercises, here is a brief recap and gallery showing what I achieved with the minimum of time spent exercising.

I am Helen Renée, an American who is married to a Brit. I was born in Minnesota and grew up in Northern Alaska after my father became an Ice Road Trucker. I went from being 40-50 lbs overweight to a contest-winning condition almost effortlessly in less than 6 months and with workout sessions lasting no longer than 10 minutes per day.

I am an isometric exercise expert instructor and champion Bikini Fitness Athlete who achieved spectacular contest-winning results after meeting my exercise scientist husband. My husband is one of the world's leading experts on isometric exercise, plant-based nutrition, and was a former coach to the 4-times World's Strongest Man, Jon Pall Sigmarsson of Iceland. I have co-authored 22 fitness books and since we share a common fascination with mysteries and the paranormal, we have co-authored a best-selling book on the subject. She is also an isometric and TRISOmetric™ exercise instructor, consultant, and instructor-trainer for TWiEA™ The World Isometric Exercise Association. www.TWiEA.com – www.HelenRenee.com

Since meeting and marrying my British husband, we have enjoyed a joyous journey together discovering the many differences between the two countries which share a common language and culture. We began writing these stories and anecdotes down and very soon had enough to produce a fun-filled and light-hearted book about what it is like Being American Married to a Brit.

The following pictures were taken in March 2015 before she started performing a daily 10 x 7-second total-body exercise isometric exercise routine.

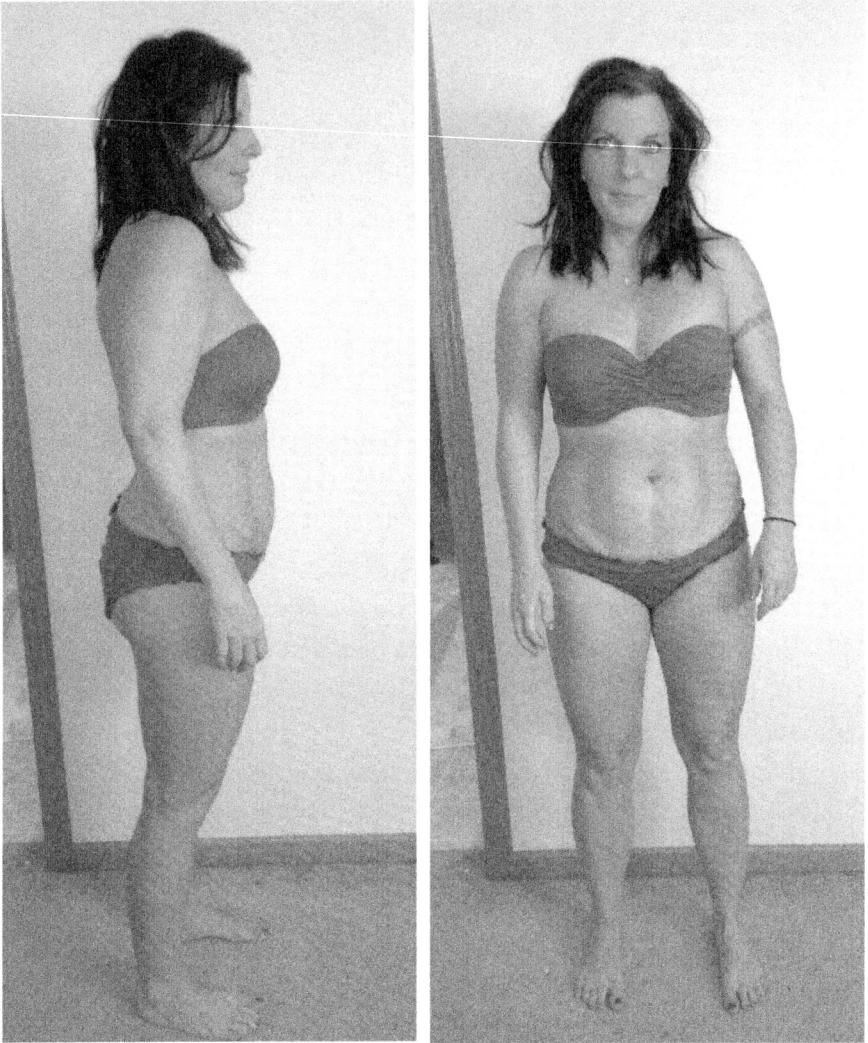

The following pictures are of me, 1-year later, in March 2016. I became a contest-winning Bikini Fitness competitor within 1-year of daily isometric exercise training lasting only minutes each day. Now, I only train using only isometric exercises because it is so effective.

I simply exercise regularly every other day and apply more intensity to each exercise than a normal person would who simply wants to get a little stronger, fitter and maintain a good overall body shape. I also eat sensibly.

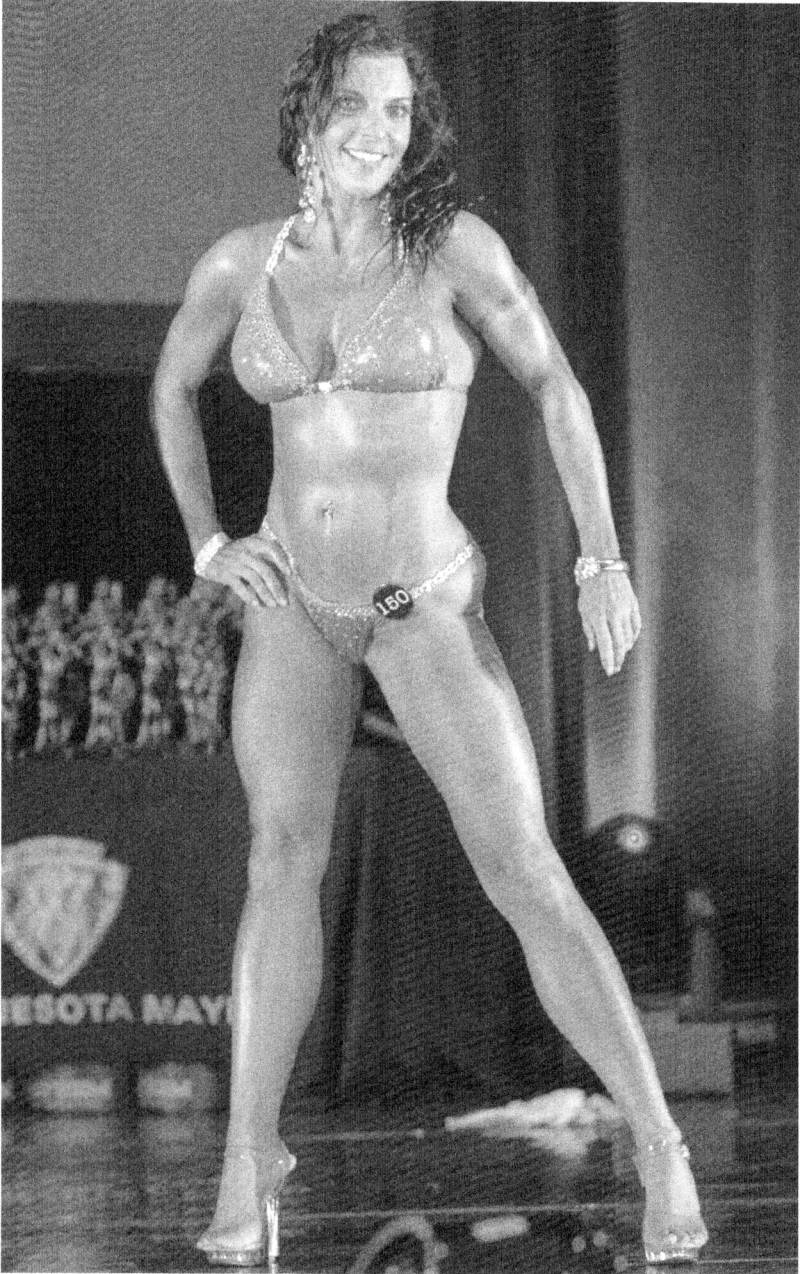

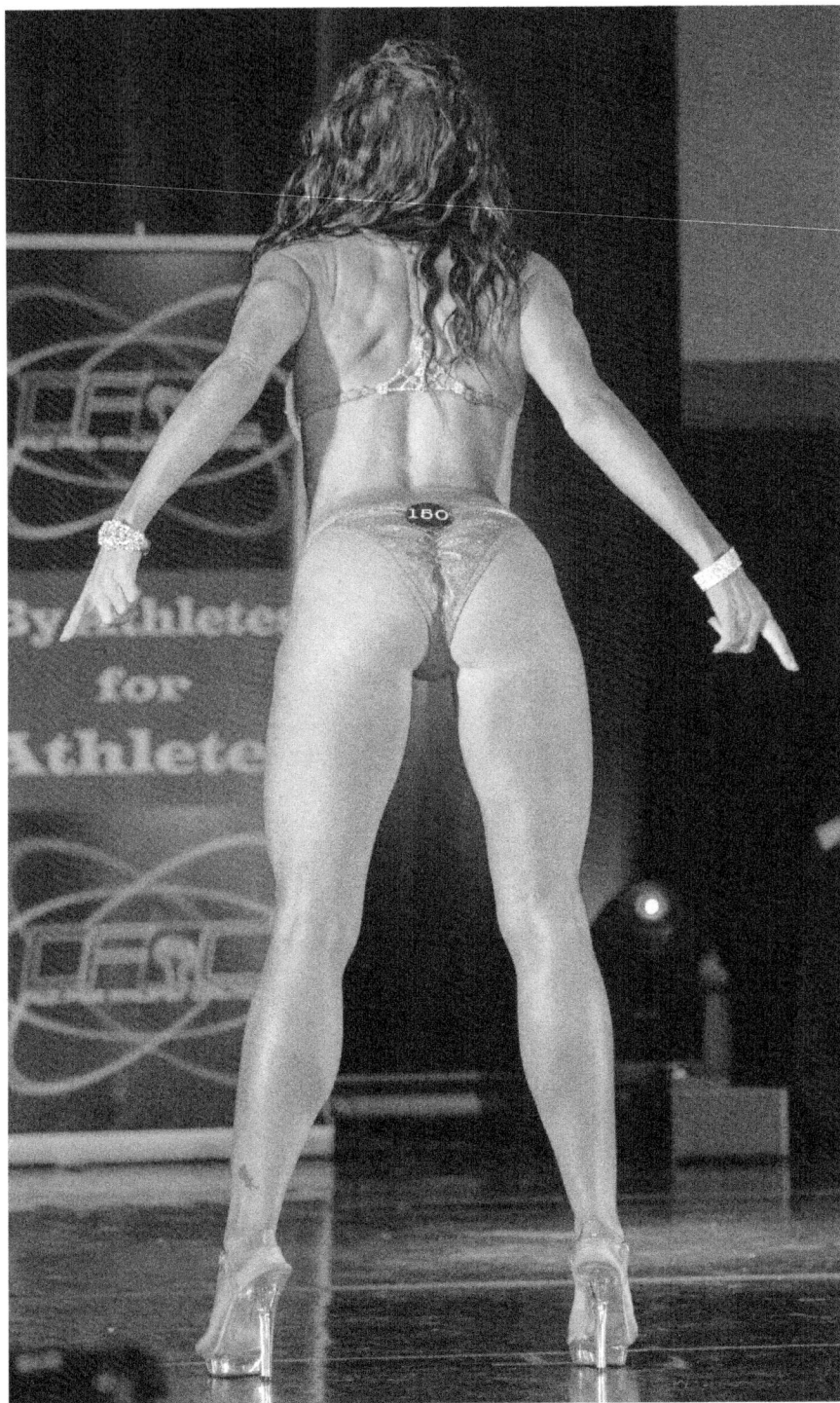

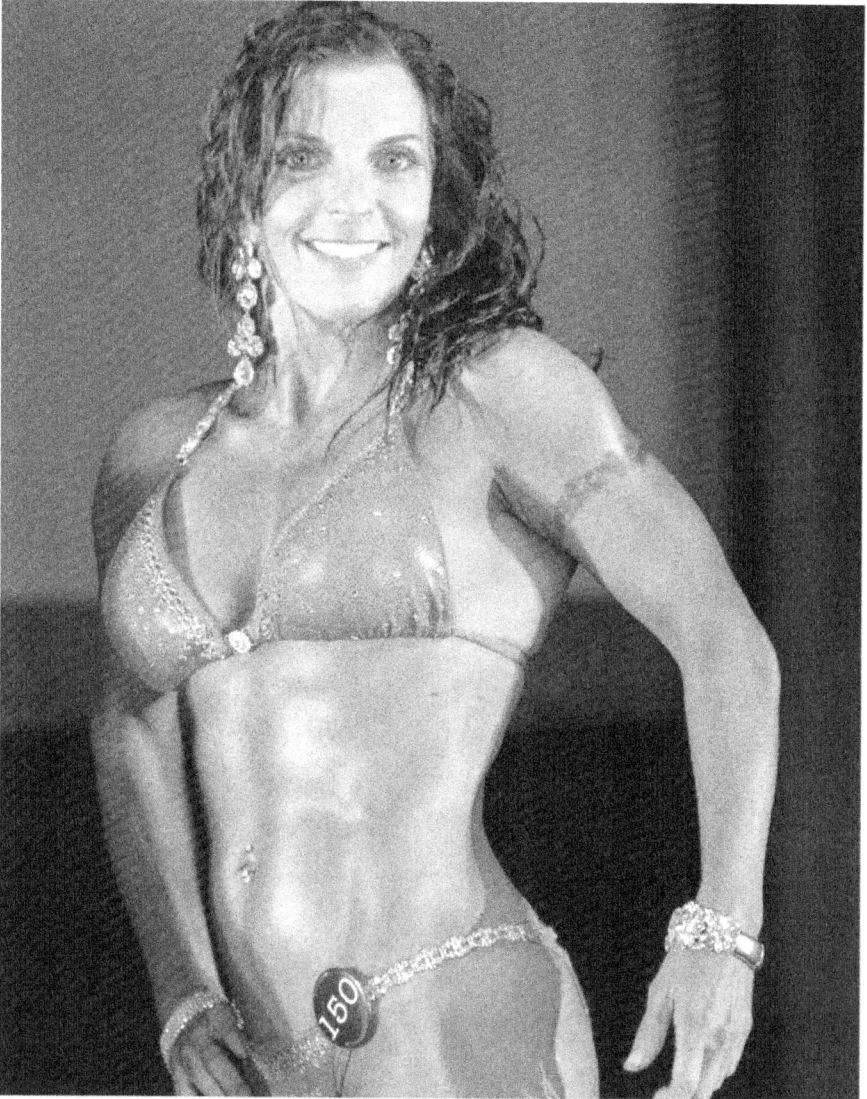

The Authors and an Isometric Experiment

Brian is my husband and co-author, and the following picture is of his arm taken in December 2016. This was after a year-long experiment to see what results could be gained through a basic high-intensity isometric exercise routine using only the minimum number of exercises.

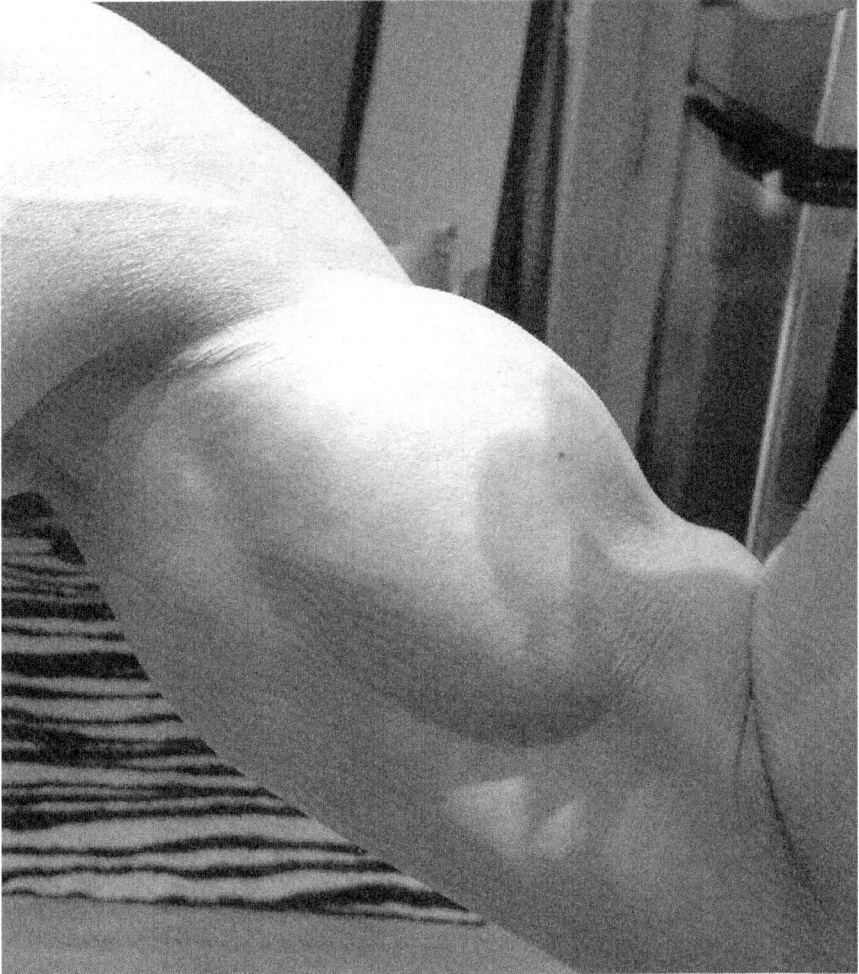

This picture of my arm was taken to record the results of the one-year isometric maintenance training experiment in December 2016. The experimental training routine allowed just 1 x 7-second isometric exercise per muscle/muscle group per day at a target level of applied force/intensity of between 75% and 80% of my estimated maximum.

For one year, starting in January 2016, he performed a daily 10 exercise x 7-second total-body isometric routine. It is common for even the most experienced athletes to count the elapsed exercise time increasingly quickly, almost in direct proportion to an increasing level of applied force/intensity. Therefore, he typically aimed to perform a 10-second isometric hold for each exercise, and this way he would always reach the desired goal of 7-seconds in good style.

His target level of intensity for each exercise was around 75-80%, slightly higher than the typically recommended average of only 2/3rds, or 66.6%. However, this still effectively meant that he exercised each of his biceps for a total of between just 21 and 30 seconds per week.

Amazingly, at the end of the year-long experiment, he achieved an improvement in both the strength and size of each arm, albeit slight. Even though he is well-versed in the science of isometrics he still found it remarkable because it was in exchange for a maximum of 30 seconds per week of exercise time. Once again, this only served to reinforce the fact that the best results are always gained through pinpoint focus, high intensity, and by never confusing activity with accomplishment.

Chapter 8. The Muscle-up For Menopause Workout

The Muscle-up for Menopause™ (MUM™) workout is a similar style to the TRISOmetric™ system combining three isometric exercises performed at different positions along the ROM (Range of Motion) of a limb/body part.

After these have been completed, a corresponding super-slow isotonic exercise is performed three times for the same muscle or muscle group.

- Remember, the MUM™ system combines three isometric exercises performed at different positions along the ROM (Range of Motion) of a limb/body part. After these have been completed, a corresponding super-slow isotonic exercise is performed for the same muscle or muscle group.
- The three isometric exercises are performed first before the isotonic exercise is performed.
- These exercises are typically performed at 60-70% of maximum intensity in each position, however, after each course change the suggested level of intensity may differ. This will be highlighted at the end of the notes section for those weeks.
- During the first two weeks of The MUM™ Course, aim for an isometric exercise intensity level of approximately 60 to 65%.
- Each of the three isometric exercise positions chosen will divide the range of motion of the limb roughly into three equal parts.
- This way a more even strength curve is developed for the muscle being exercised.
- This takes advantage of the strength gain overlap area of + and − 20% around the point of isometric exercise chosen.
- Before you begin the full isometric contraction part of the exercise, take between two and three additional seconds to perform Dynamic Flexation™ to help you properly engage the muscles and joints.

- Similarly, at the end of each isometric exercise, do the same in reverse as you disengage from the exercise over a period of between two and three seconds.
- Perform only one seven second isometric exercise contraction in each of the three selected positions.
- Do not start counting the isometric exercise time until you have fully applied the desired level of intensity to the exercise.
- There should be no longer than 10 seconds of rest time between each isometric exercise.
- Once all three isometric exercises have been completed, with a maximum rest time of 10 seconds since the end of the last isometric exercise, then a corresponding isotonic exercise is performed to exercise the same muscles/muscle group.
- All exercises can be performed with no equipment as freehand (bodyweight only) isometrics or callisthenics, or with strong climbing rope, a towel, a Bullworker®, a Steel Bow®, an Iso-Bow®, an Iso-gym®, a doorway pull-up bar, push-up handles or with weights/resistance machines. The choice is yours according to your ability and the equipment you have available to you.
- The method of performing the isotonic exercise must always be in a super-slow style which takes 10 to 12 seconds to perform one repetition in each direction.
- This means that each repetition should take 10 to 12 seconds for the concentric or lifting phase where the muscles shorten, and another 10 to 12 seconds for the eccentric or lowering phase where the muscles lengthen. This will engage and activate many more muscle fibres than if the same exercise were performed in a faster exercise style.
- It may help to use a countdown timer on your mobile phone that is visible while you exercise.
- Remember, that it is quite easy to perform an isotonic exercise too quickly, however, it is hard to perform an isotonic exercise too slowly.
- Always breathe naturally and never hold your breath when exercising.

- If it takes 10 to 12 seconds to perform each phase of the super-slow isotonic portion of the exercise, then take as many as 10 to 12 breaths (or more) in and out during each phase.
- Counting the number of breaths in and out as one second of elapsed time will help you to count more efficiently while exercising, and to help keep your breathing natural and steady.
- Perform The MUM™ Course workouts on Monday / Wednesday / Friday of each week with at least one full day of rest between workout sessions and two days of rest over each weekend.
- If needed, take an extra day of rest between workout sessions because rest and recovery are vital. However, try not to take more than two days of rest between workout sessions.

For an absolute beginner, please feel free to start out completing each month with the mid-position hold only.

Once you feel comfortable, you may progress to include the mid-position hold and upper position hold.

Again, once you have mastered these two holds, you may complete the full three-position isometric holds (mid, upper, and lower positions) and then include the isotonic movement.

Suggested Equipment

1) Climbing rope or similar.

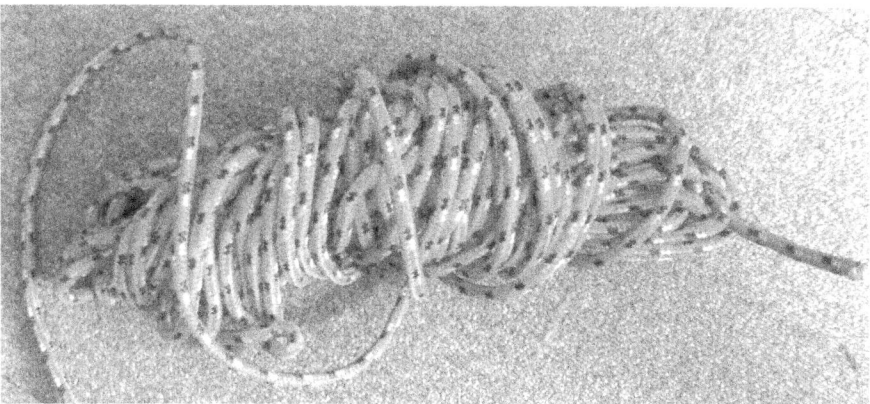

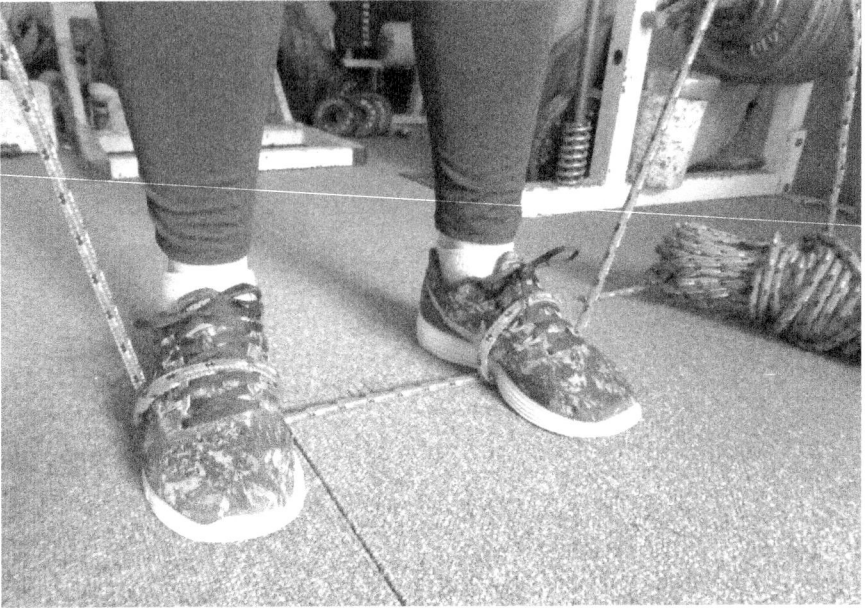

2) Doorway pull-up bar.

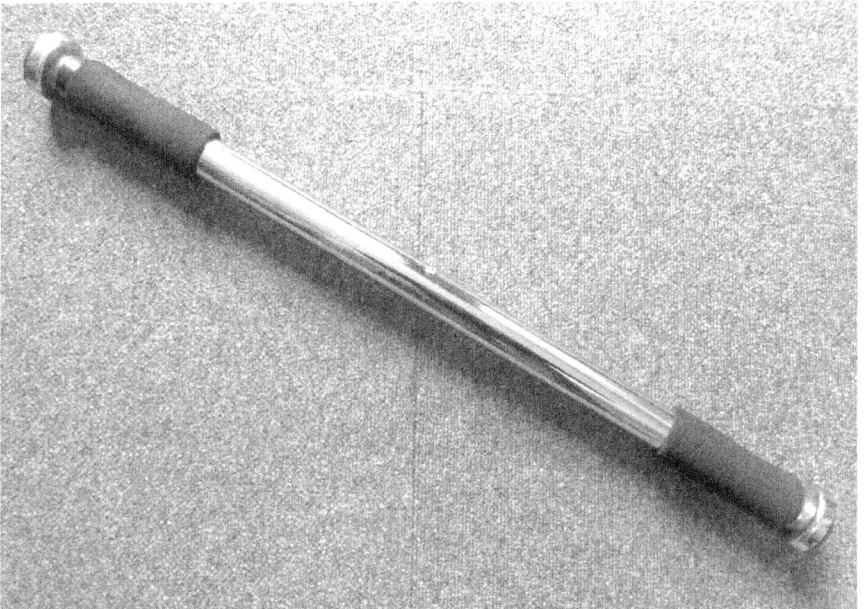

3) Beach towel.

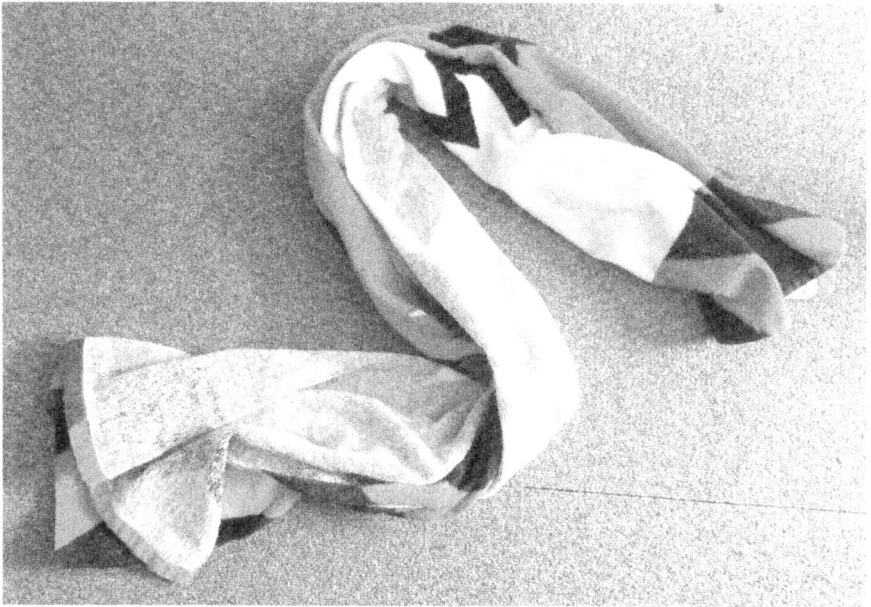

4) 2 x Iso-Bows®.

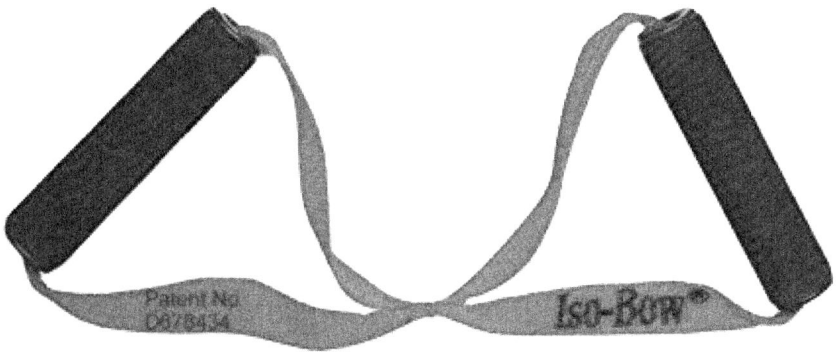

5) Push-up handles.

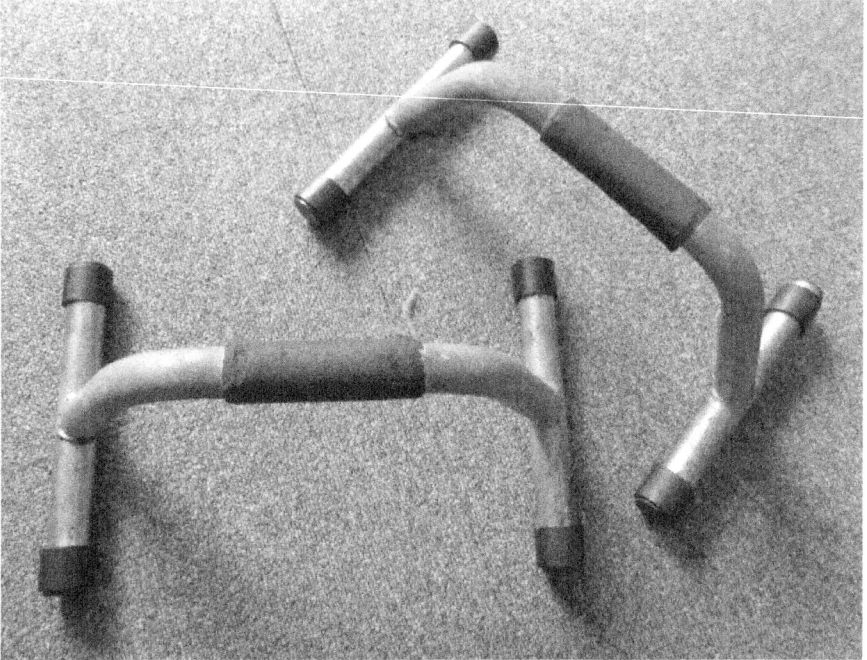

Optional push-up handles to increase the
ROM (Range Of Motion)

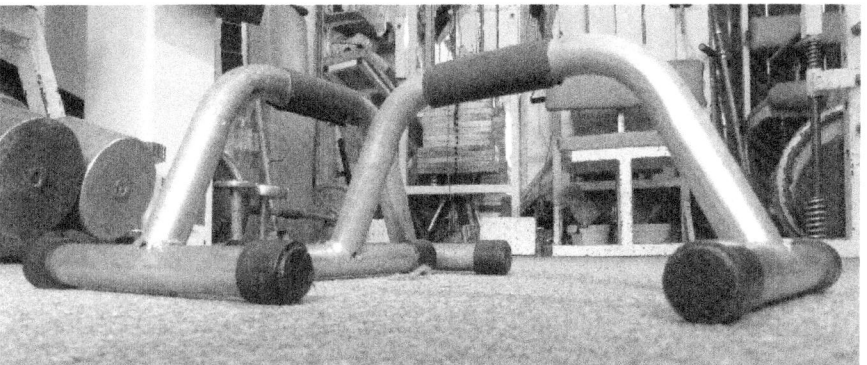

The Muscle-up For Menopause™ (MUM™) Course - 1st Month at a Glance

1. Legs - Upper
   a. Isometric
      i. Isometric Wall Hack Squat (Triple Position Hold)
   b. Isotonic
      i. The Isotonic Squat
2. Legs - Calf's
   a. Isometric
      i. Isometric Calf Double Leg Wall Push (Triple Position Hold)
   b. Isotonic
      i. Isotonic Double Heel Raise
3. Chest
   a. Isometric
      i. Resisted Push-up (From Feet) (Triple Position Hold) (Rope / Iso-Gym® Strap / Towel)
   b. Isotonic
      i. Push-ups (From Feet)
4. Shoulders
   a. Isometric
      i. Lateral Pull-Apart (Triple Position Hold) (Rope / Iso-Bow® / Towel / Hands)
   b. Isotonic
      i. Pendulum Lateral Raise (Rope / Iso-Bow® / Towel / Hands)
5. Triceps & Biceps
   a. Isometric
      i. Biceps and Triceps Press-Curl (Left Side) (Triple Position Hold)
   b. Isotonic
      i. Biceps and Triceps Press-Curl (Left Side) (Triple Position Hold)

6. Triceps & Biceps
   a. Isometric
      i. Biceps and Triceps Press-Curl (Right Side) (Triple Position Hold)
   b. Isotonic
      i. Biceps and Triceps Press-Curl (Right Side) (Triple Position Hold)
7. Abdominals
   a. Isometric
      i. Bent-Knee Trunk Crunch (Triple Position Hold) (Bodyweight Resisted)
   b. Isotonic
      i. Bent-Knee Crunch
8. Back - Lower
   a. Isometric
      i. Bent Leg Deadlift (Rope / Iso-Bow® / Towel) (Triple Position Hold)
   b. Isotonic
      i. Floor Hyperextensions
9. Forearms
   a. Isometric
      i. Water Bottle Grip (Single, Double or Triple Position Hold)
   b. Isotonic
      i. NONE - This is an isometric-only exercise
10. Back - Upper
   a. Isometric
      i. Sitting Seated Row (Triple Position Hold) (Rope / Iso-Bow® / Towel / Hands)
   b. Isotonic
      i. Sitting Seated Row (Rope / Iso-Bow® / Towel / Hands)

1. Legs Upper
A) Isometric Wall Hack Squat (Triple Position Hold)

First, decide each of the angles you will assume when performing the three successive isometric exercises. Then decide if you will use any equipment or not, and if so, what it will be. If you are going to use any equipment then deploy and test it in advance of beginning both the isometric and isotonic exercise phases for this body part, even if it will only be used for just one of the phases.

Place the back of your torso flat against a solid wall or door. If using a door, make sure that you use the side that closes back into the frame so that it cannot accidentally open or be opened as you exercise. Position your feet approximately shoulder-width apart in a medium stance with the toes slightly pointed out. Bend your legs to assume the first isometric exercise angle, keep your back flat against the wall/door, your head upright and place your arms in a comfortable position. Attempt to straighten your legs as if you are trying to simultaneously push and lift the wall or door using your thighs as the primary driving force.

Gradually apply pressure using Dynamic Flexation™ until you have applied the approximate desired target level of intensity, then begin the first isometric exercise.

When you perform an isometric exercise never hold your breath. Always breathe deeply and naturally, which will be about 10 full breaths in and out at a rate of about 1 second per full breath. Perform each exercise for no less than 7 seconds, and no longer than 10. Try not to rest between each exercise for longer than 10 seconds, which should allow enough time to recover while getting into the next position.

Once you have assumed the next isometric exercise angle, perform the exercise in the same way as the previous one, and then perform the third angle isometric exercise in the same way. With the triple isometric portion of the exercise completed, try to rest for no longer than 10 seconds before performing the isotonic phase.

135

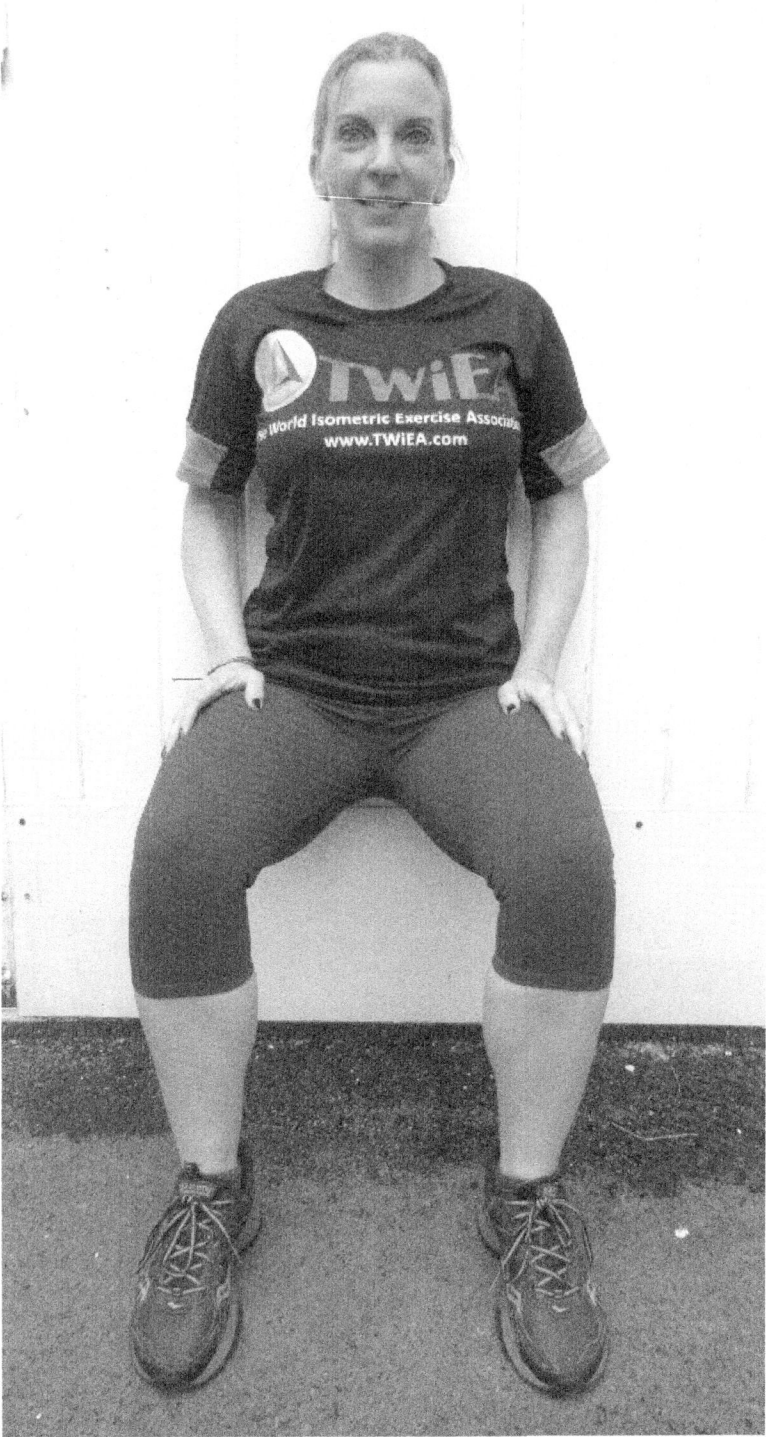

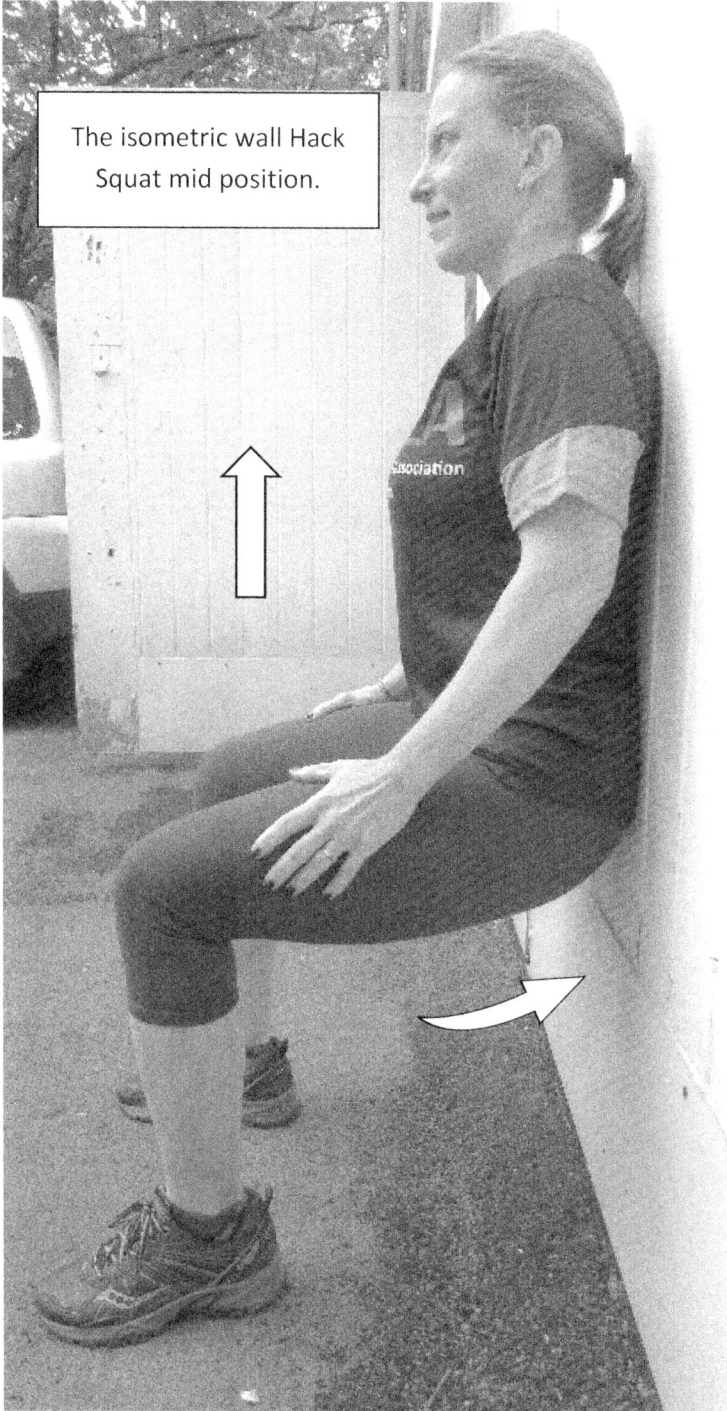

The isometric wall Hack Squat mid position.

The isometric wall Hack Squat lower position.

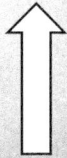

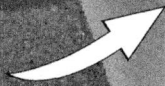

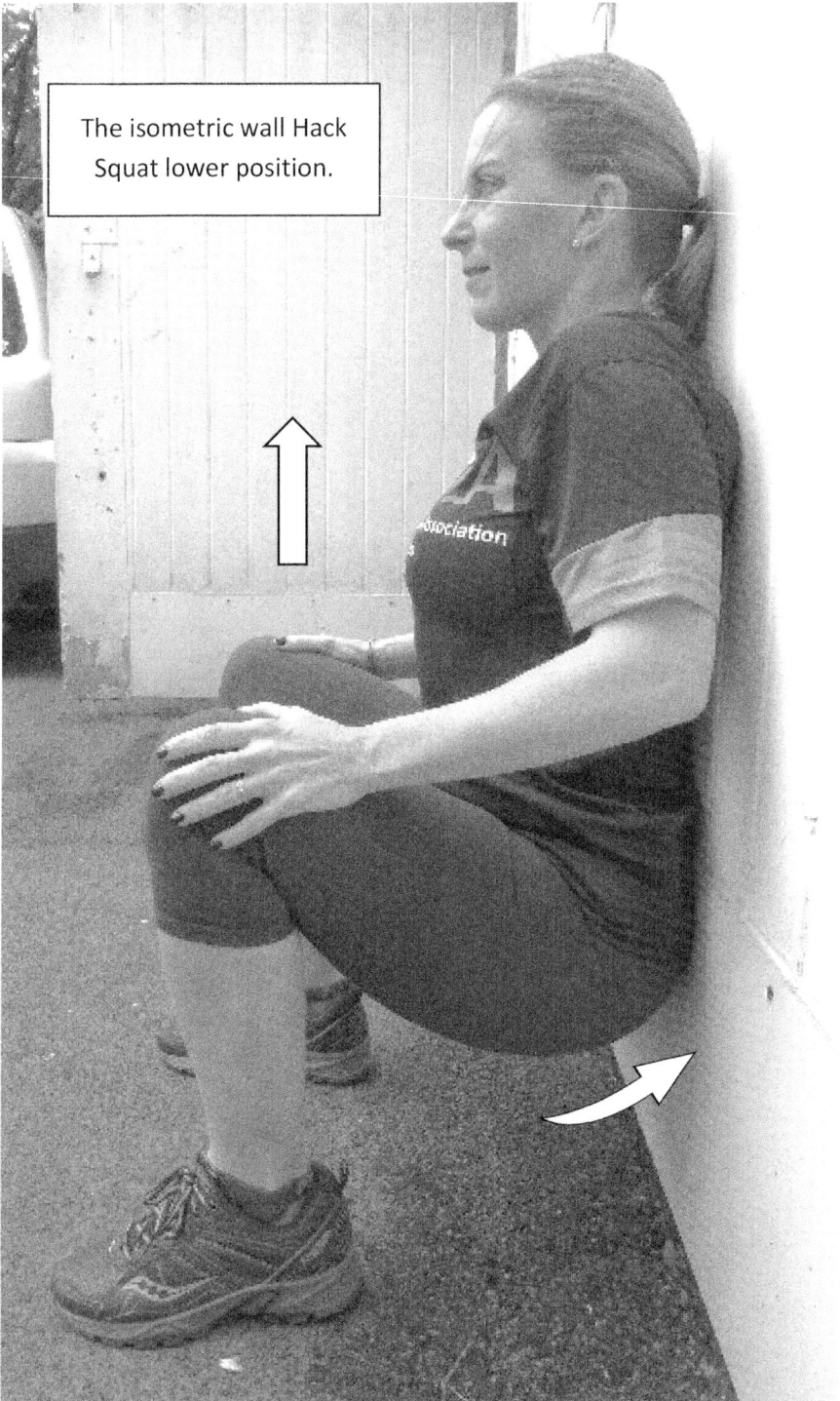

The isometric wall Hack Squat upper position.

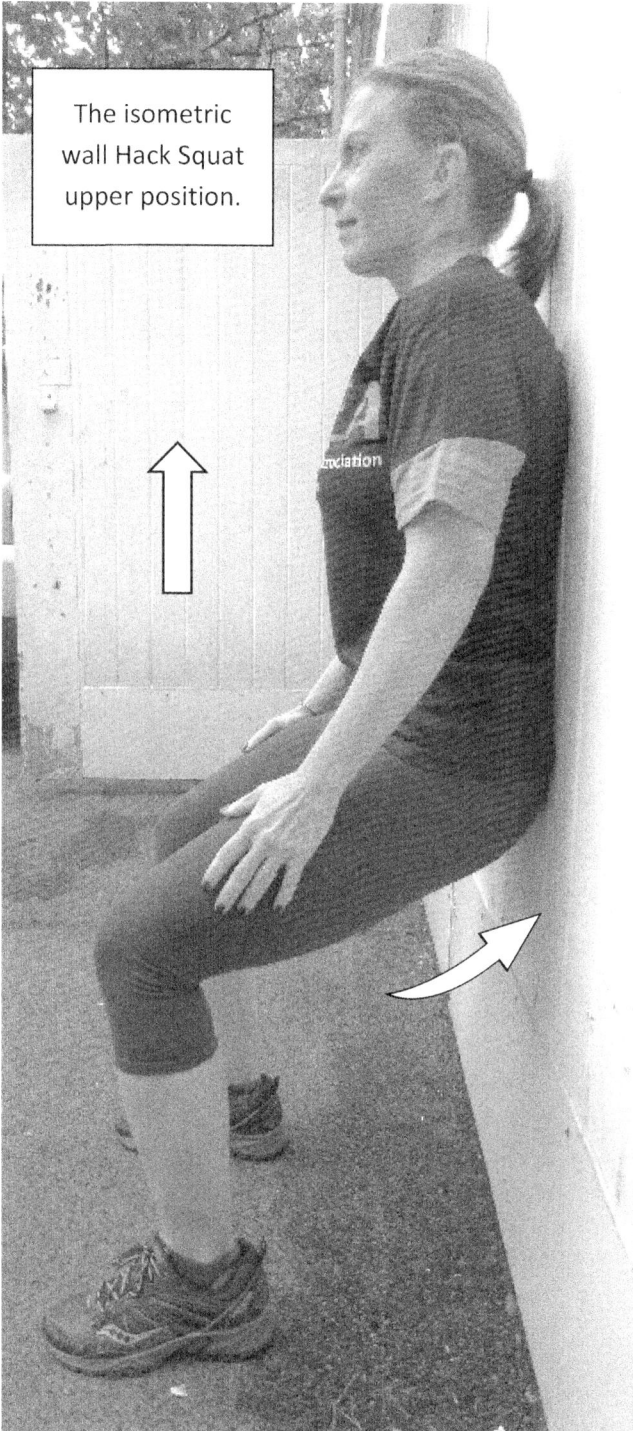

B) The Isotonic Squat

Place your feet approximately shoulder-width apart and bend your knees to squat down until your thighs are parallel to the floor. As you do so, keep your back straight, head upright and bend forward only from the hip.

To perform a correct squat in the lowest position the front of the knees should make an imaginary straight line perpendicular with the toes to the front. If your knees are past the imaginary line, then you are placing undue stress on the knees.

When you reach the lowest point of the squat, pause for a second before rising back to the starting position.

The exercise should be performed in super-slow style with each portion of the exercise (eccentric and concentric) taking between 10 and 12 seconds to complete. This makes it extremely challenging by any standards.

Never hold your breath, and a suggested method of breathing during super-slow repetitions is to breathe in and out one full breath for each second of elapsed time.

Aim to perform one set of three repetitions, but do not be surprised if you can only manage one at super-slow speed. If this is your limit, even only one repetition performed at super-slow speed will deliver all the results you desire. Do not sacrifice good exercise style and true super-slow speed in exchange for a greater number of repetitions at a faster speed.

You will gradually increase the number of repetitions you can perform by following the science and adhering to a strict exercise style and good technique.

If needed, use a chair, wall, or any other solid object to help with your balance.

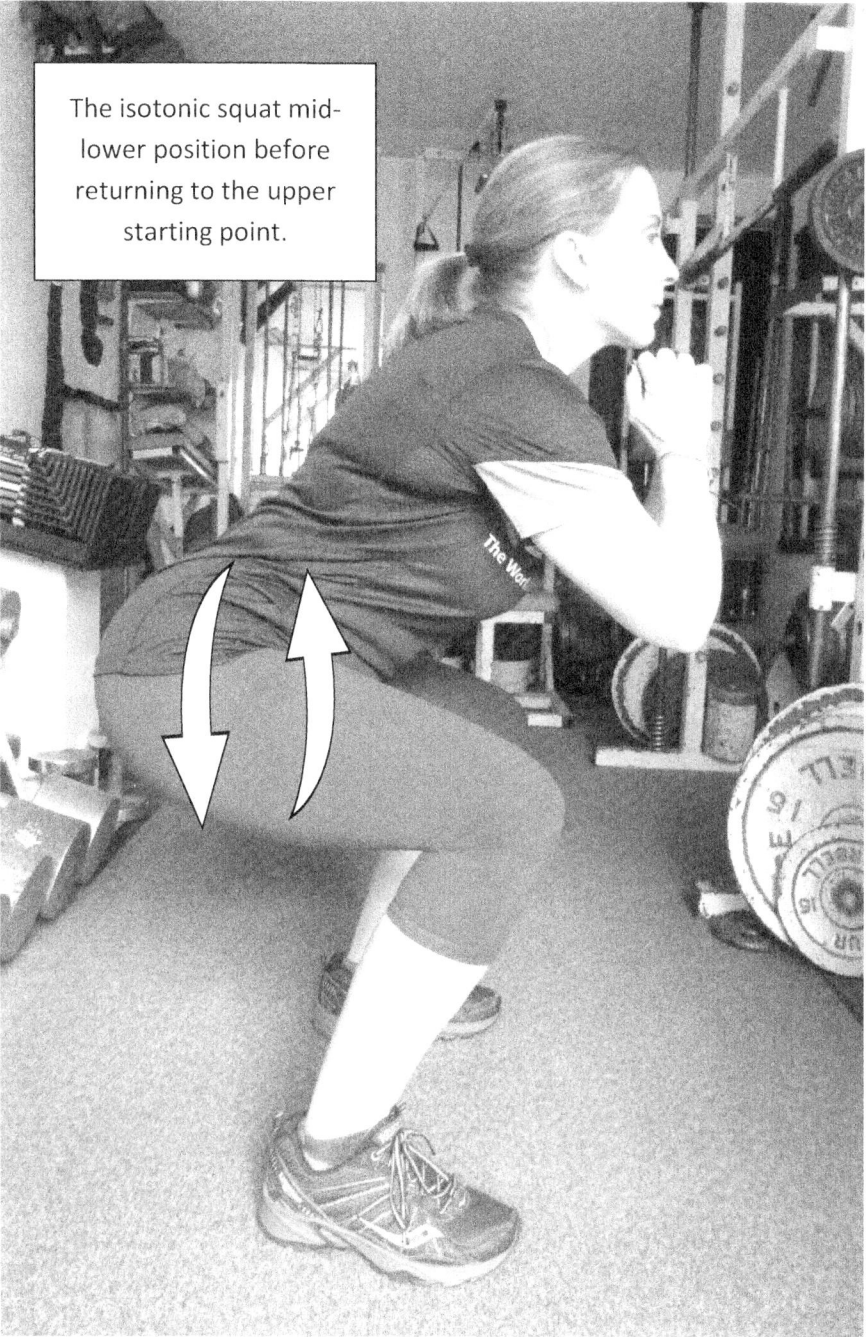

The isotonic squat mid-lower position before returning to the upper starting point.

Notes About Foot and Knee Positions During Thigh/Leg Exercises:

If you position your feet at approximately shoulder-width apart in a medium stance with the toes slightly pointed out it will evenly engage your overall thigh muscles, a wider stance with knees apart will engage the inner thigh muscles more, while a close foot and knees together position will engage the outer thigh muscles more.

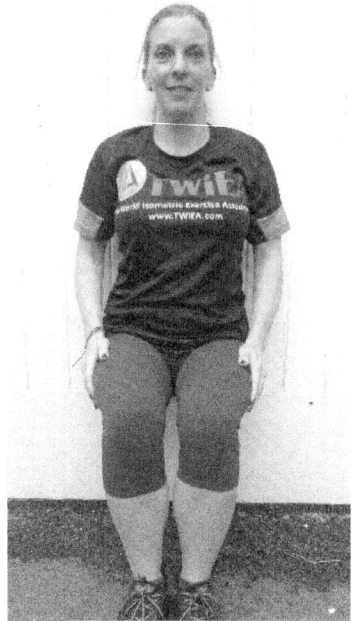

Knees Narrow: Emphasis on Outer Thighs

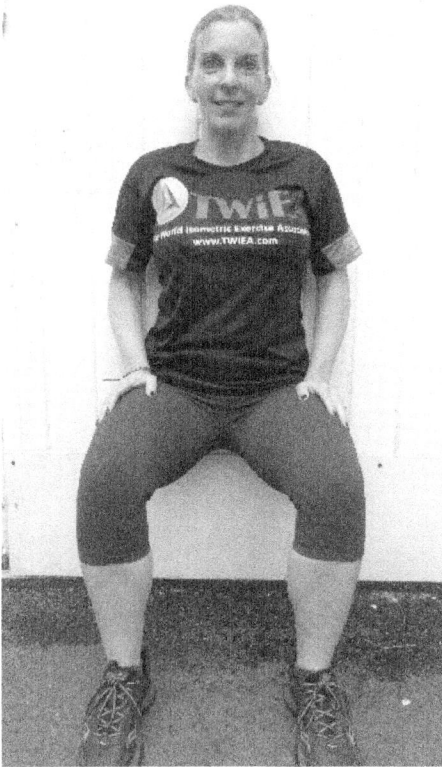

Knees Neutral: Emphasis on Mid Thighs

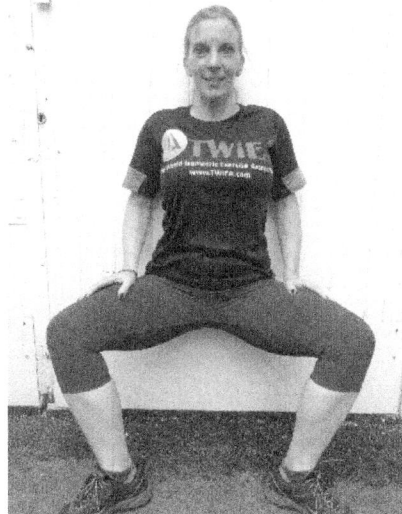

Knees Wide: Emphasis on Inner Thighs

2. Legs - Calf's
A) Isometric Calf Double Leg Wall Push (Triple Position)

First, decide each of the angles you will assume when performing the three successive isometric exercises. There is a limited range of motion in the heel raise exercise so this will require a little thought and preplanning. Then decide if you will use any equipment or not, and if so, what it will be.

If you are going to use any equipment then deploy and test it in advance of beginning both the isometric and isotonic exercise phases for this body part, even if it will only be used for just one of the phases. Face a wall or solid door which closes away from you so it cannot accidentally open or be opened during the exercise. Place your feet roughly shoulder-width apart, with your legs straight and toes facing forwards.

Lean slightly forward towards the wall or door and place both hands flat on the surface at approximately shoulder height as if you intend to push it over. Attempt to raise the heels of each foot to the correct position for the first isometric exercise. Gradually apply pressure using Dynamic Flexation™ until you have applied the approximate desired target level of intensity, then begin the first isometric exercise.

When you perform an isometric exercise never hold your breath. Always breathe deeply and naturally, which will be about 10 full breaths in and out at a rate of about 1 second per full breath. Perform each exercise for no less than 7 seconds, and no longer than 10. Try not to rest between each exercise for longer than 10 seconds, which should allow enough time to recover while getting into the next position.

Once you have assumed the next isometric exercise angle, perform the exercise in the same way as the previous one, and then perform the third angle isometric exercise in the same way.

With the triple isometric portion of the exercise completed, try to rest for no longer than 10 seconds before performing the isotonic phase.

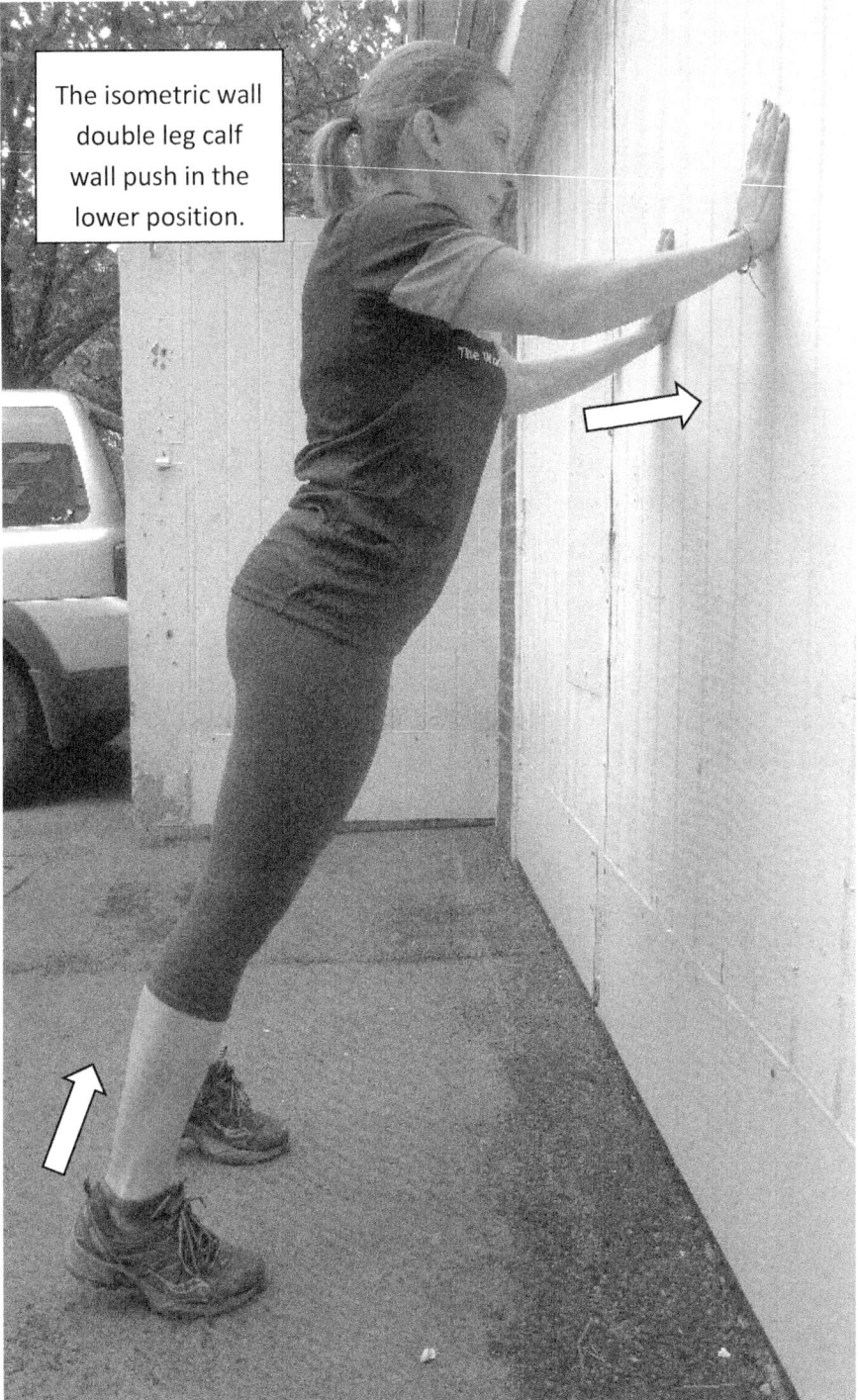

The isometric wall double leg calf wall push in the lower position.

The three positions of the isometric calf wall push.

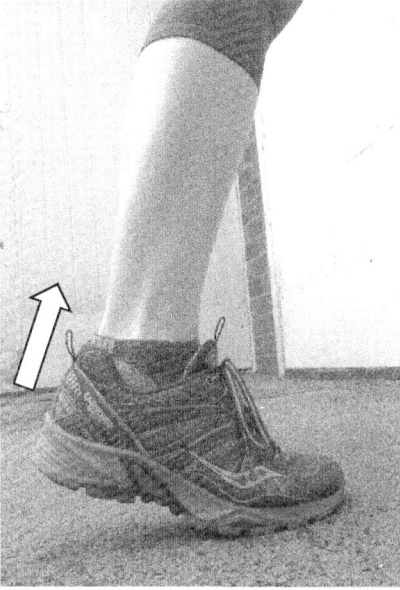

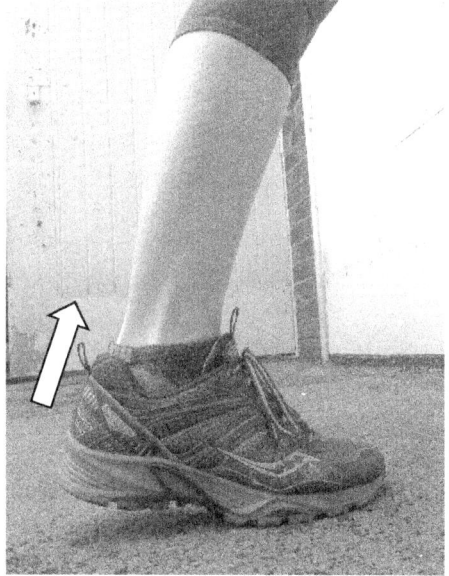

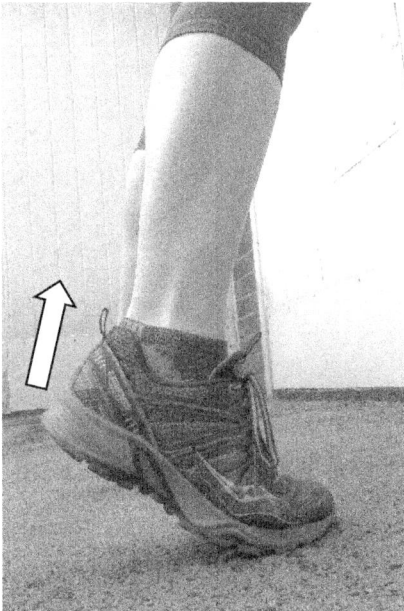

B) Isotonic Double Heel Raise

In the same position, keep your fingertips on the wall or door to aid your balance.

In this position, slowly raise both heels from the floor to the highest point you can reach, pause for a second and then return to the starting position, pause, and repeat.

The exercise should be performed in super-slow style with each portion of the exercise (eccentric and concentric) taking between 10 and 12 seconds to complete. This makes it extremely challenging by any standards.

Since there is only a limited range of motion that can be performed, it will feel almost like you are performing a sequence of many multi-point short duration isometric exercises as you raise and lower the heels. This is precisely what it should feel like to gain maximum benefit.

Never hold your breath, and a suggested method of breathing during super-slow repetitions is to breathe in and out one full breath for each second of elapsed time.

Aim to perform one set of three repetitions, but do not be surprised if you can only manage one at super-slow speed. If this is your limit, even only one repetition performed at super-slow speed will deliver all the results you desire.

Do not sacrifice good exercise style and true super-slow speed in exchange for a greater number of repetitions at a faster speed.

You will gradually increase the number of repetitions you can perform by following the science and adhering to a strict exercise style and good technique.

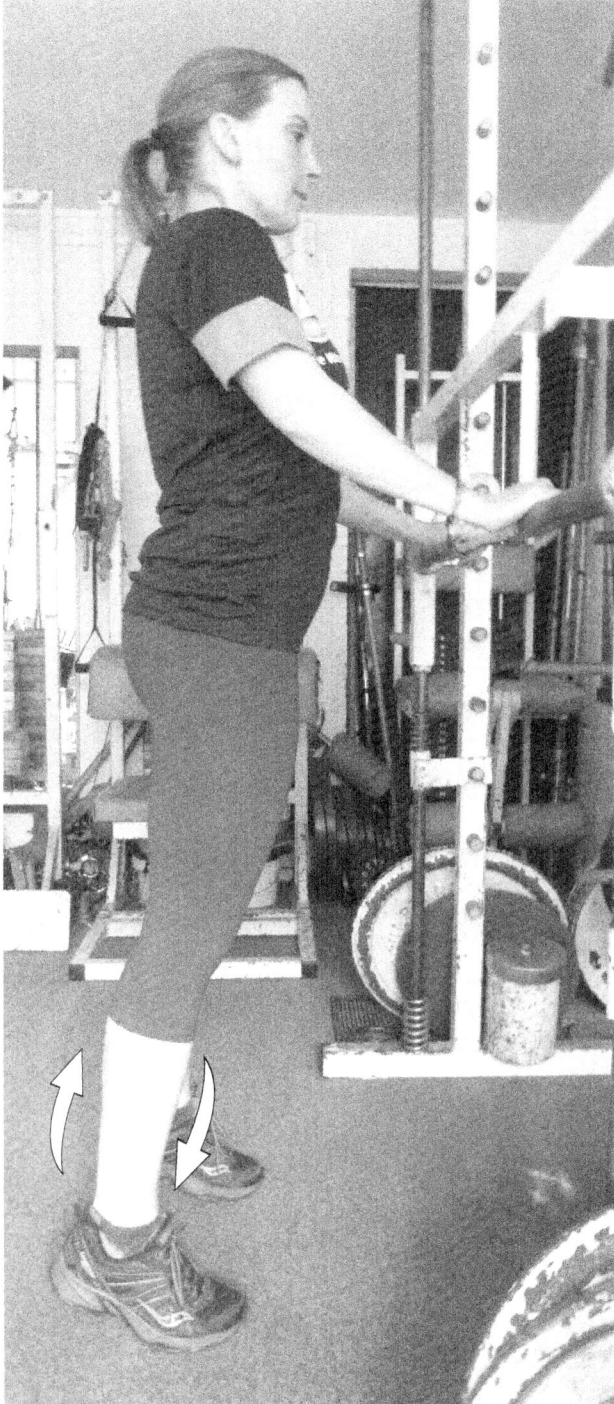

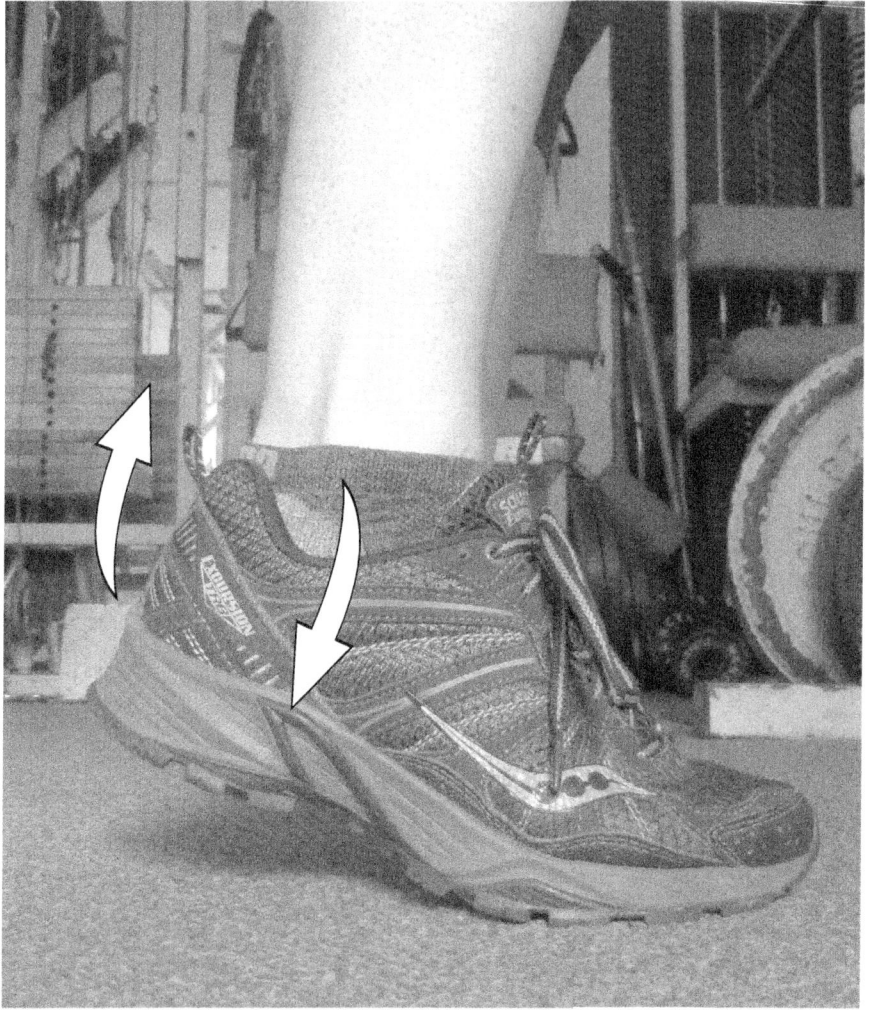

3. Chest

A) Isometric *Resisted Push-up (From Feet) (Triple Position Hold)* (Rope / Iso-Gym® Strap / Towel)

First, decide each of the angles you will assume when performing the three successive isometric exercises. Decide if you will use any equipment or not, and if so, what it will be. We will assume that you will use a rope for this description. Place and hold a strong climbing rope around your upper back so that you can loop it around each hand at the correct length for each of the three isometric exercise positions. Kneel on an exercise mat and place the palms of your hands flat on the floor slightly wider than shoulder-width apart, elbows at about 45 degrees of abduction (away from the body), fingers pointing forward, and with your legs extended behind you as far as possible to rest on your feet.

When in the first resisted isometric push-up position with your bodyweight resting on the palms of your hands. Gradually apply pressure using Dynamic Flexation™ until you have applied the approximate desired target level of intensity, then begin the first isometric exercise. When you perform an isometric exercise never hold your breath. *Always breathe deeply and naturally*, which will be about 10 full breaths in and out at a rate of about 1 second per full breath. Perform each exercise for no less than 7 seconds, and no longer than 10. Try not to rest between each exercise for longer than 10 seconds, which should allow enough time to recover while getting into the next position.

Once you have assumed the next isometric exercise angle, perform the exercise in the same way as the previous one, and then perform the third angle isometric exercise in the same way. With the triple isometric portion of the exercise completed, try to rest for no longer than 10 seconds before performing the isotonic phase.

NOTE: Push-up handles can be used to greatly increase the ROM (Range Of Motion) and difficulty of this exercise, and they work equally well for both the isometric and isotonic phases.

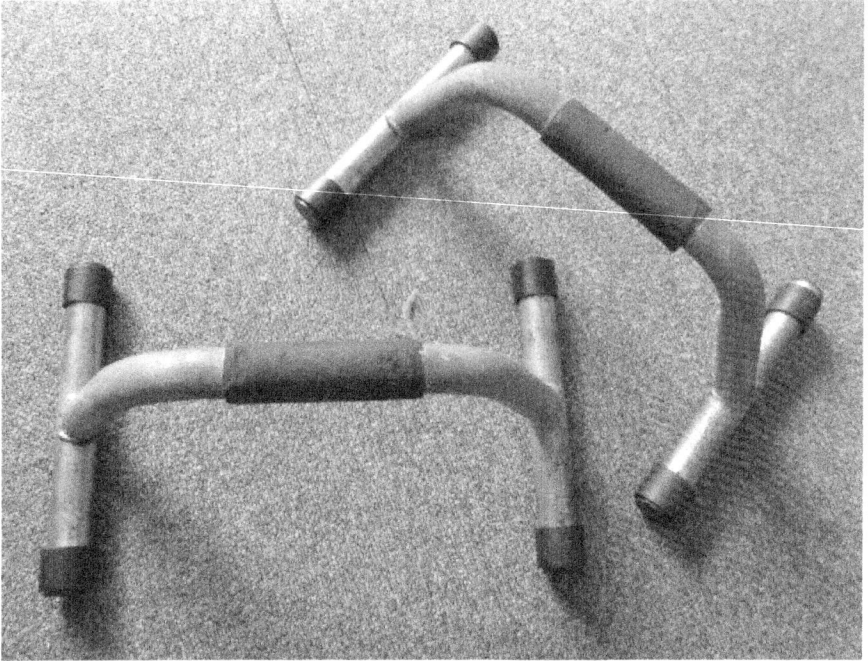

Optional push-up handles to increase the
ROM (Range Of Motion)

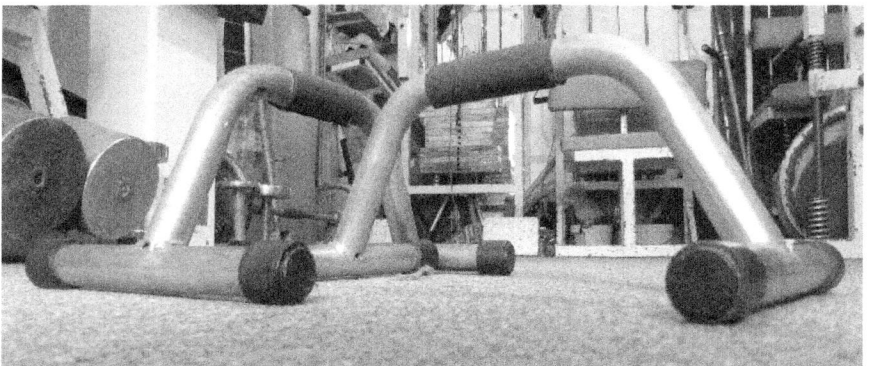

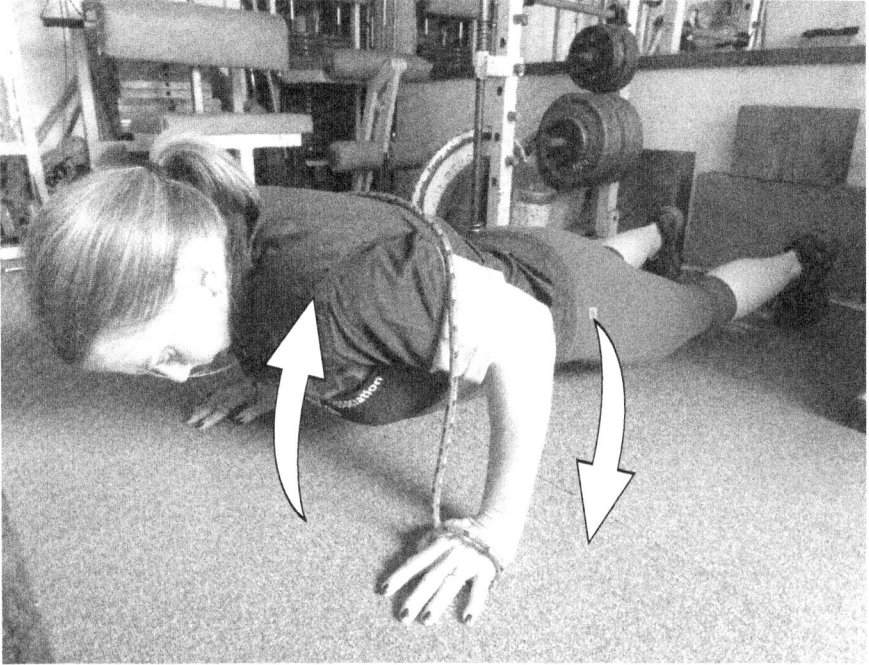

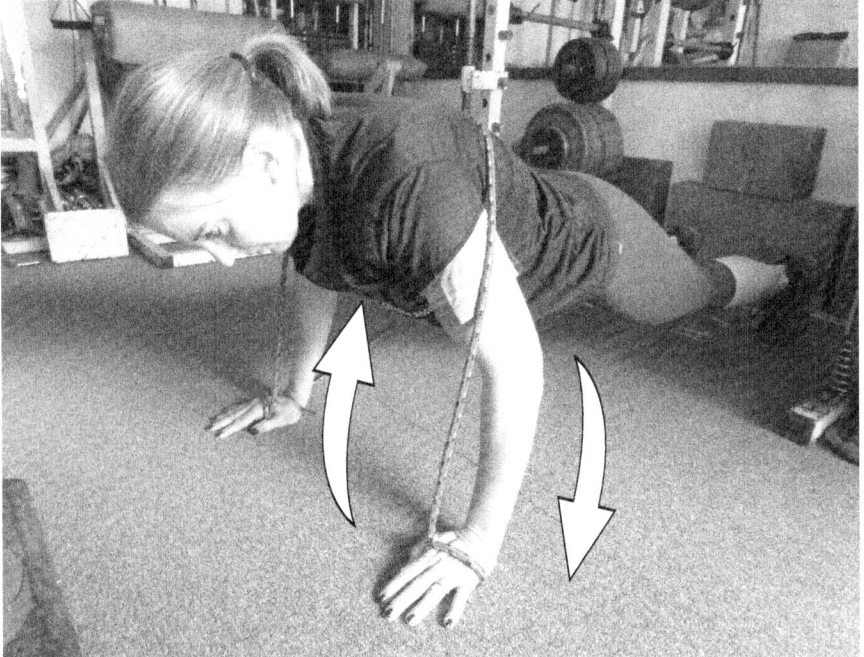

NOTE: When performing either the isometric or isotonic chest press exercise if you cannot perform it by supporting your body on your hands and feet, then perform it by supporting your body on your hands and knees to make it easier.

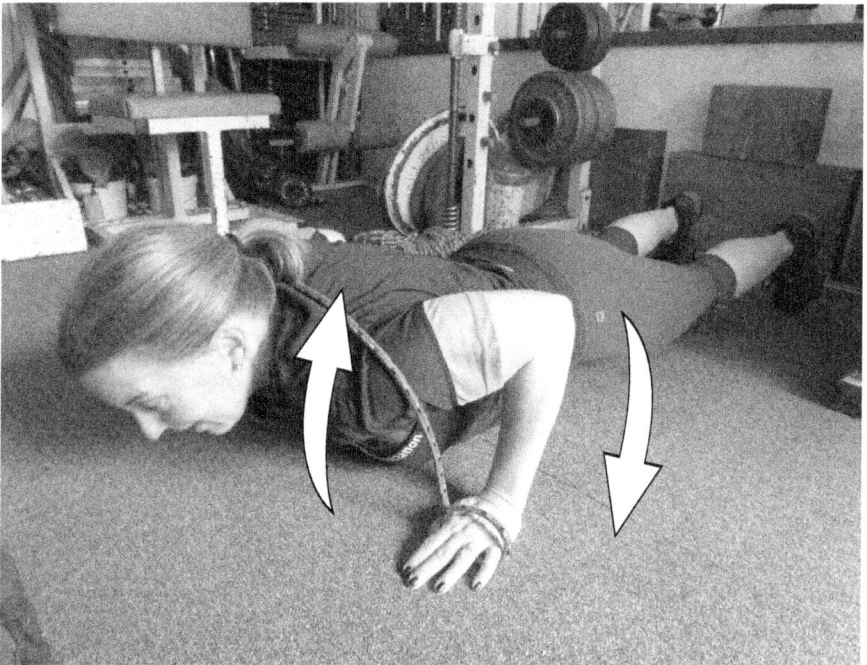

B) Isotonic Push-ups (From Feet or Knees)

Kneel on an exercise mat and place the palms of your hands flat on the floor slightly wider than shoulder-width apart, your elbows at about 45 degrees of abduction (away from the body), your fingers pointing forward, and with a foot/knee position of choice back behind the hips. If you are able, then perform the push-ups from the feet instead of the knees. However, when you reach the point that you cannot perform another push up in this way, then perform the next one from the knees until you can no longer perform any more repetition, or when you have reached 12 repetitions.

When performing push-ups from the knees, then the further back you position your knees, the harder the exercise will be to perform, and the further forward the knee position, the easier the exercise will be to perform. When in the traditional push-up position with your bodyweight resting on the palms of your hands with your arms straight. Keeping your back straight and abdominal muscles flexed to support you, lower yourself towards the floor and stop a faction before touching it, pause, then return to the starting position.

The exercise should be performed in super-slow style with each portion of the exercise (eccentric and concentric) taking between 10 and 12 seconds to complete. This makes it extremely challenging by any standards. Never hold your breath, and a suggested method of breathing during super-slow repetitions is to breathe in and out one full breath for each second of elapsed time.

Aim to perform one set of three repetitions, but do not be surprised if you can only manage one rep at super-slow speed. If this is your limit, even only one performed at super-slow speed will deliver all the results you desire. Do not sacrifice good exercise style and true super-slow speed in exchange for a greater number of repetitions at a faster speed. You will gradually increase the number of repetitions you can perform by following the science and adhering to a strict exercise style and good technique.

NOTE 1: The hardest exercise position is when performing push-ups with suspended on the hands and feet.

As the exercise becomes increasingly challenging, drop down onto the knees to make it easier. This way you will perform more repetitions.

When performing push-ups from the knees, then the further back you position your knees, the harder the exercise will be to perform, and the further forward the knee position, the easier the exercise will be to perform.

NOTE 2: Push-up handles can be used to greatly increase the ROM (Range Of Motion) and difficulty of this exercise, and they work equally well for both the isometric and isotonic phases.

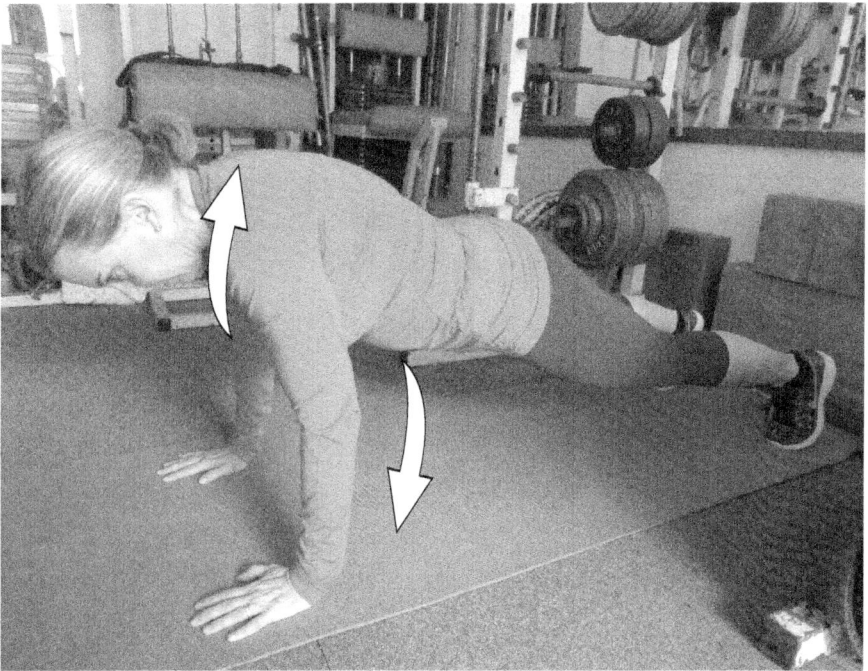

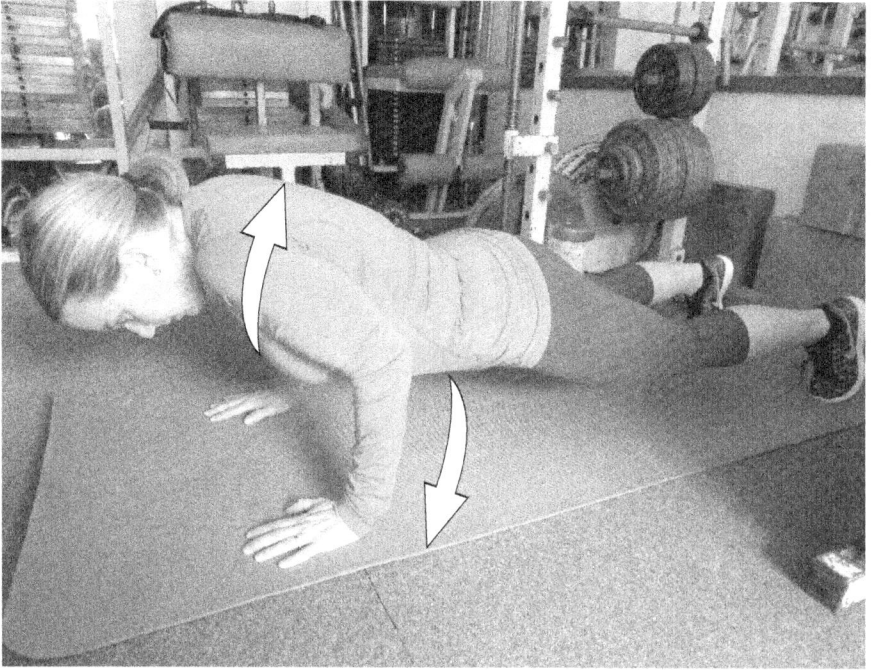

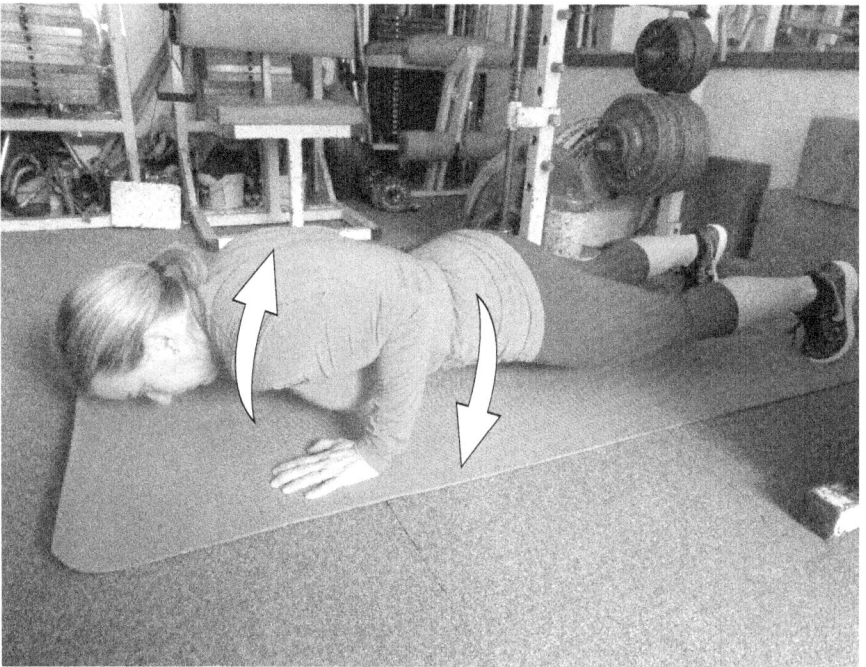

4. Shoulders

A) Isometric Lateral Pull-Apart (Triple Position Hold) (Rope / Iso-Bow® / Towel / Hands)

First, decide each of the angles you will assume when performing the three successive isometric exercises. Then decide if you will use any equipment or not, and if so, what it will be. If you are going to use any equipment then deploy and test it in advance of beginning both the isometric and isotonic exercise phases for this body part, even if it will only be used for just one of the phases.

When using no equipment, stand upright and interlock your fingers and hands in front of you at arm's length at hip level. Bend both arms slightly in a no-lock elbow position.

If you are using rope or a towel, then make sure you grip it securely. You can loop the rope around hour hands if needed. An Iso-Bow® or similar will provide you with the best grip.

Attempt to raise the arms sideways in an arc motion using your shoulder muscles as the driving force to perform the deltoid exercise to the correct position for the first isometric exercise.

Gradually apply pressure using Dynamic Flexation™ until you have applied the approximate desired target level of intensity, then begin the first isometric exercise.

When you perform an isometric exercise never hold your breath. Always breathe deeply and naturally, which will be about 10 full breaths in and out at a rate of about 1 second per full breath. Perform each exercise for no less than 7 seconds, and no longer than 10.

Try not to rest between each exercise for longer than 10 seconds, which should allow enough time to recover while getting into the next position.

Once you have assumed the next isometric exercise angle, perform the exercise in the same way as the previous one, and then perform the third angle isometric exercise in the same way.

With the triple isometric portion of the exercise completed, try to rest for no longer than 10 seconds before performing the isotonic phase.

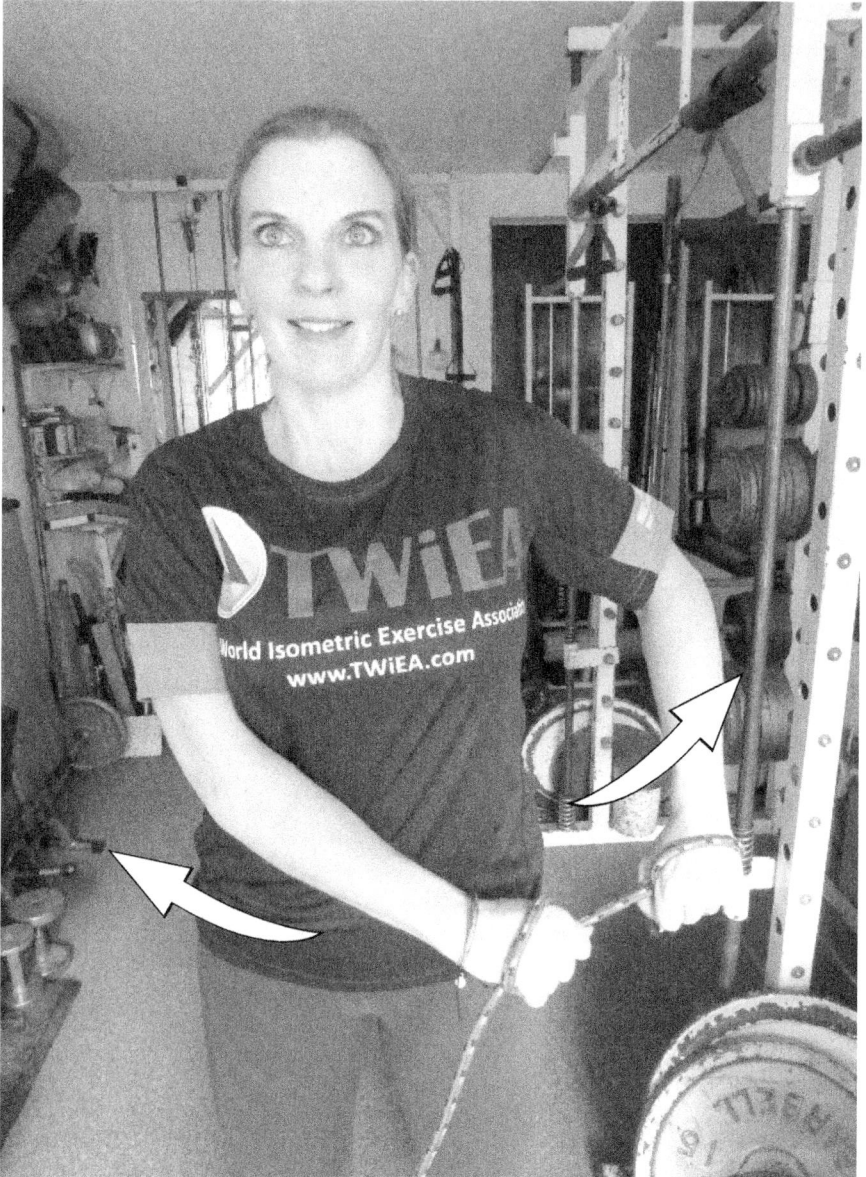

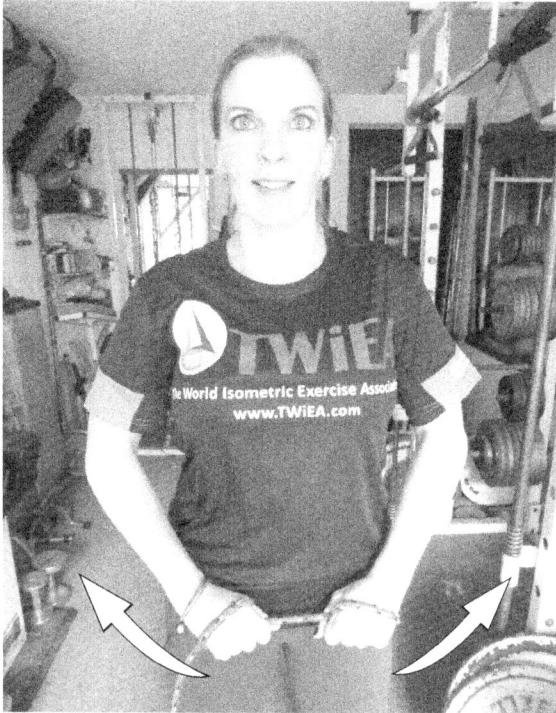

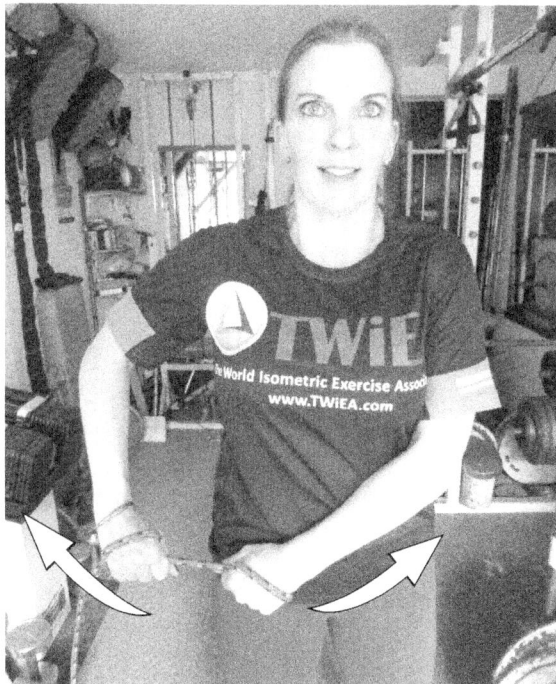

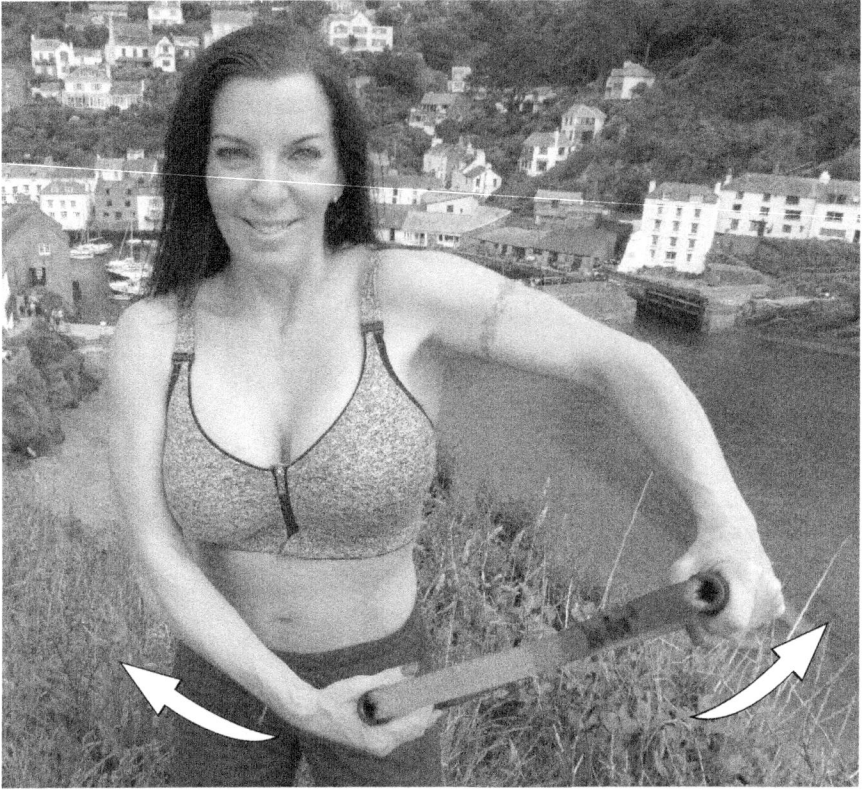

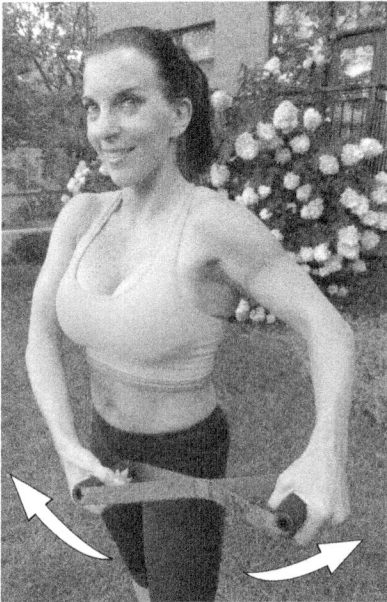

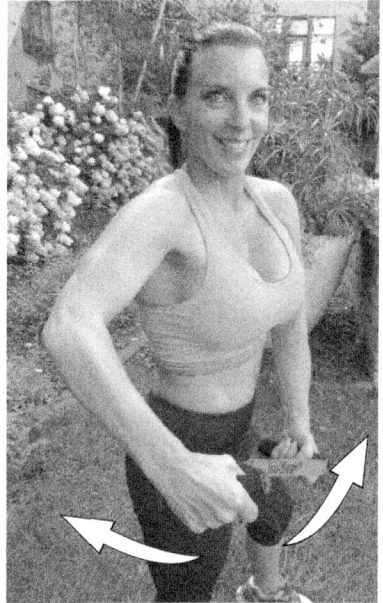

B) Isotonic Pendulum Lateral Raise (Rope / Iso-Bow® / Towel / Hands)

When using no equipment, stand upright and interlock your fingers and hands in front of you at arm's length at hip level. Bend both arms slightly in a no-lock elbow position.

If you are using rope or a towel, then make sure you grip it securely. You can loop the rope around hour hands if needed. An Iso-Bow® or similar will provide you with the best grip.

In this position, gradually apply pressure using Dynamic Flexation™ as you attempt to raise the arms using your shoulder muscles as the driving force to perform the deltoid exercise first to one side then the other in a pendulum arc motion. Your upper body should remain completely immobile in a fixed upright position throughout the exercise

The exercise should be performed in super-slow style with each portion of the exercise (eccentric and concentric) taking between 10 and 12 seconds to complete. This makes it extremely challenging by any standards.

Never hold your breath, and a suggested method of breathing during super-slow repetitions is to breathe in and out one full breath for each second of elapsed time.

Aim to perform one set of between 3 repetitions, but do not be surprised if you can only manage one repetition at super-slow speed. If this is your limit, even only one repetition performed at super-slow speed will deliver all the results you desire.

Do not sacrifice good exercise style and true super-slow speed in exchange for a greater number of repetitions at a faster speed.

You will gradually increase the number of repetitions you can perform by following the science and adhering to a strict exercise style and good technique.

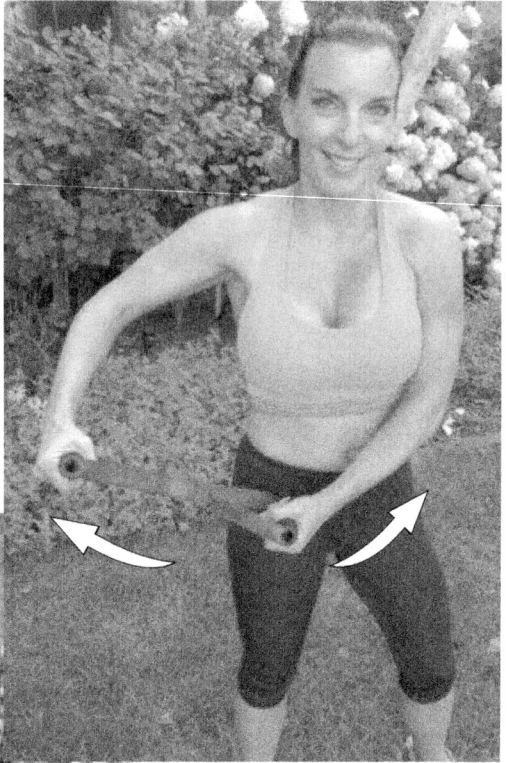

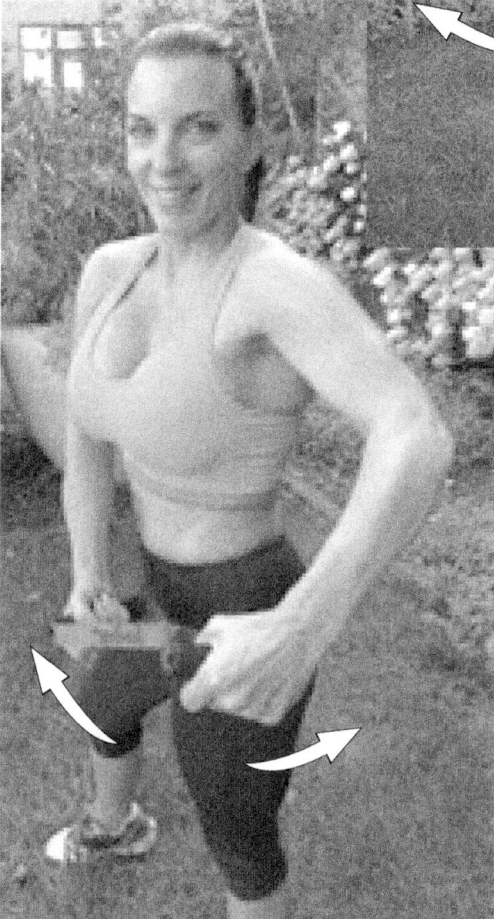

6. Triceps and Biceps (Right)

A) Isometric Biceps and Triceps Press-Curl (Left and Right Side) (Triple Position Hold)

First, decide each of the angles you will assume when performing the three successive isometric exercises. Then decide if you will use any equipment or not, and if so, what it will be.

If you are going to use any equipment then deploy and test it in advance of beginning both the isometric and isotonic exercise phases for this body part, even if it will only be used for just one of the phases.

When using no equipment, stand upright and interlock your fingers and hands in front of you at arm's length at hip level. Bend both arms slightly in a no-lock elbow position.

If you are using rope or a towel, then make sure you grip it securely. You can loop the rope around hour hands if needed. An Iso-Bow® or similar will provide you with the best grip.

The biceps and triceps dual resistance technique will exercise the biceps muscles on one arm, while at the same time exercising the triceps muscles on the other arm.

One arm, with the palms of the hands facing downwards, interlocks hands with the other arm with palms facing upwards. Both arms and elbows must always remain close to the body, with elbows bent to allow the muscles to be exercised properly.

Attempt to raise the arms sideways in an arc motion using your shoulder muscles as the driving force to perform the deltoid exercise to the correct position for the first isometric exercise.

Gradually apply pressure using Dynamic Flexation™ until you have applied the approximate desired target level of intensity, then begin the first isometric exercise.

Perform all the isometric and isotonic exercise phases for one side of the boys/set of muscles before progressing to exercise the remaining muscles in the same way.

When you perform an isometric exercise never hold your breath. Always breathe deeply and naturally, which will be about 10 full breaths in and out at a rate of about 1 second per full breath.

Perform each exercise for no less than 7 seconds, and no longer than 10. Try not to rest between each exercise for longer than 10 seconds, which should allow enough time to recover while getting into the next position.

Once you have assumed the next isometric exercise angle, perform the exercise in the same way as the previous one, and then perform the third angle isometric exercise in the same way.

With the triple isometric portion of the exercise completed, try to rest for no longer than 10 seconds before performing the isotonic phase.

NOTE: Some people prefer to perform this exercise with the hands positioned roughly along the midline at the front of the body, or with alternate hands/arms at opposing sides of the body.

Both methods are fine, and it is more important to find a position that works best for you.

Never allow your wrists to bend backwards during any exercise as this reduces the level of intensity that can be applied.

Also, remember to change from palms up to palms down on each hand/side to exercise the biceps and triceps of both arms.

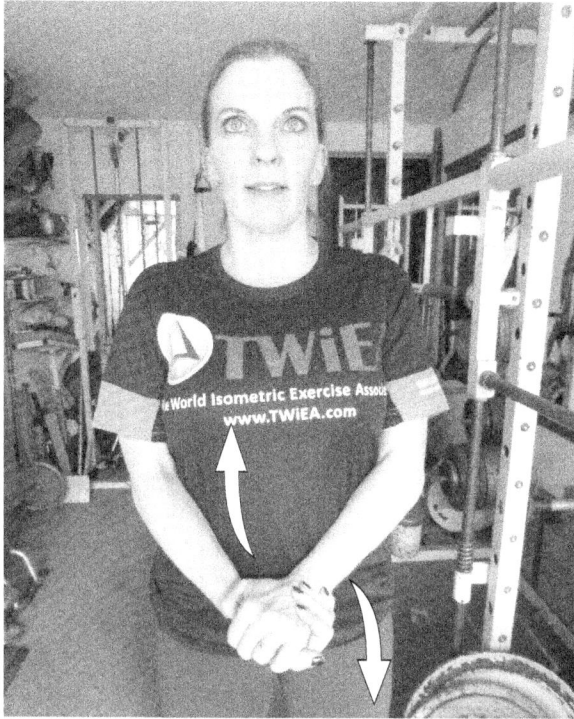

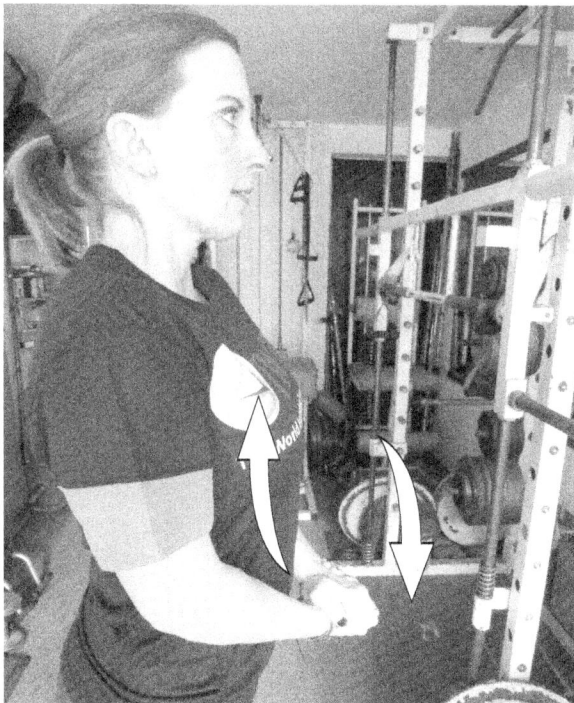

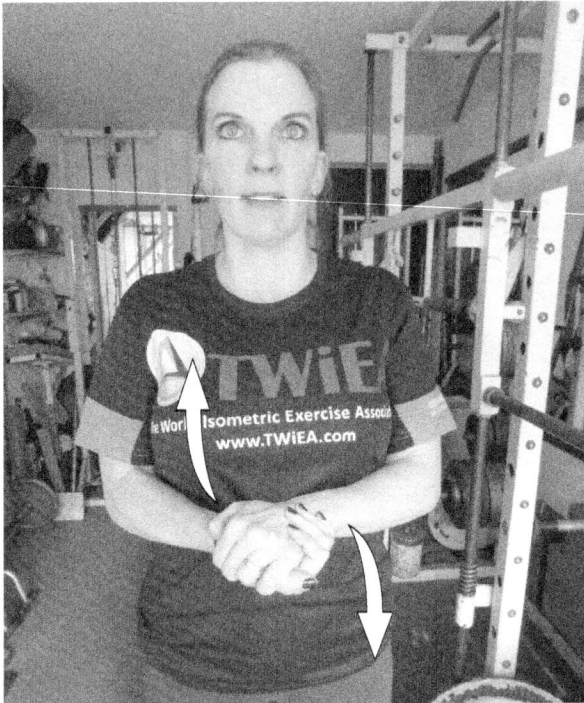

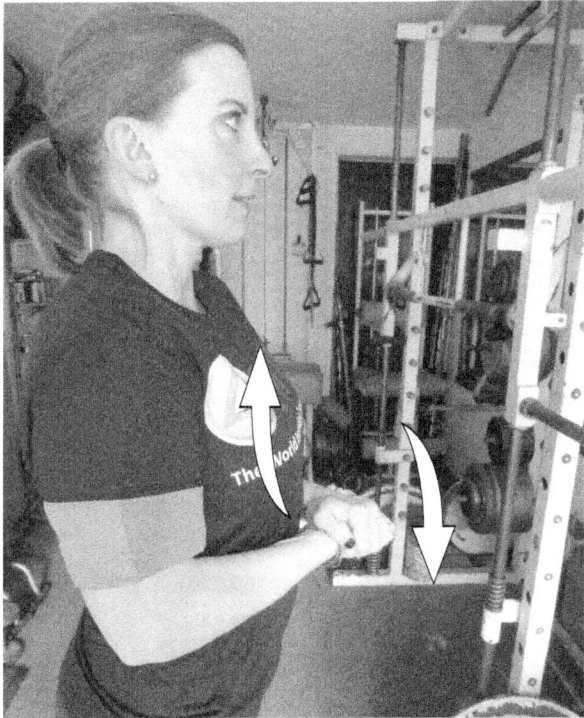

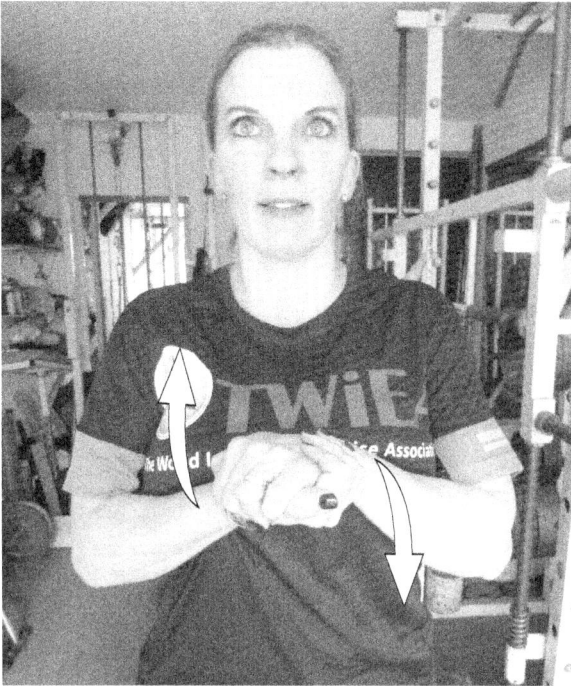

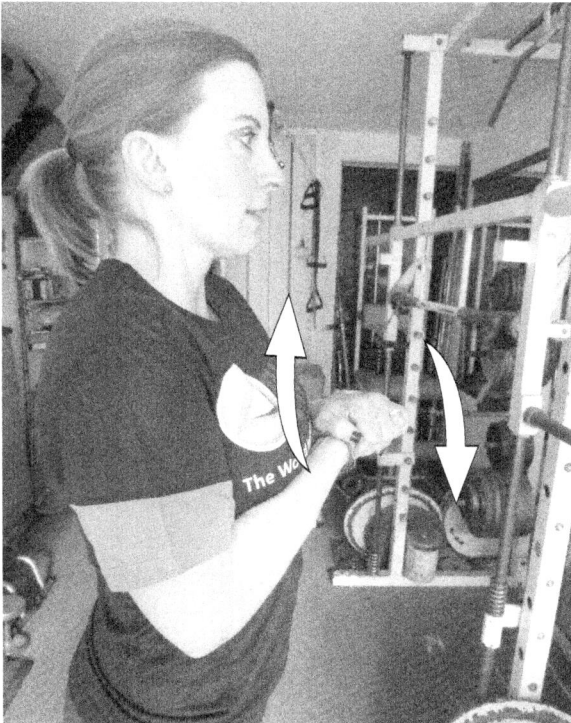

B) Isotonic Biceps and Triceps Press-Curl (Left and Right Side)

When using no equipment, stand upright and interlock your fingers and hands in front of you at arm's length at hip level in the same way as when you began the isometric phase. Bend both arms slightly in a no-lock elbow position.

One arm, with the palms of the hands facing downwards, interlocks hands with the other arm with palms facing upwards. Both arms and elbows must always remain close to the body, with elbows bent to allow the muscles to be exercised properly.

In this position, gradually apply pressure using Dynamic Flexation™ as you attempt to apply the desired level of intensity as you perform a biceps curl with one arm and triceps press with the other arm simultaneously.

The exercise should be performed in super-slow style with each portion of the exercise (eccentric and concentric) taking between 10 and 12 seconds to complete. This makes it extremely challenging by any standards.

Never hold your breath, and a suggested method of breathing during super-slow repetitions is to breathe in and out one full breath for each second of elapsed time.

Aim to perform one set of three repetitions, but do not be surprised if you can only manage one repetition at super-slow speed. If this is your limit, even only one repetition performed at super-slow speed will deliver all the results you desire.

Do not sacrifice good exercise style and true super-slow speed in exchange for a greater number of repetitions at a faster speed. You will gradually increase the number of repetitions you can perform by following the science and adhering to a strict exercise style and good technique.

7. Abdominals- (Bodyweight Resisted)
A) Isometric Bent-Knee Crunch (Triple Position Hold)

First, decide each of the angles to perform the three successive isometric exercises. Then decide if you will use any equipment or not, and if so, what. If you are, then deploy and test it in advance of beginning both exercise phases, even if it will only be used for just one of the phases. Lie back on the floor with both knees bent and your feet flat on the floor about shoulder-width apart. Place your arms with clenched fists together in front of your chest and stomach, so your fists sit just under your chin to support your neck and head. Contract your abdominals and curl your body upwards as if you are slowly peeling it from the floor fractionally with your shoulders leading. It should feel as though you are beginning to curl yourself and wrap around a large ball. Keep your lower back flat on the floor, and the highest point of the exercise is always just before the lower back is about to rise. There is a limited range of motion in this exercise and never allow yourself to begin performing a full sit up. Once you are in the first isometric exercise position, hold at that point. In this position, gradually apply pressure using Dynamic Flexation™ until you have applied the approximate desired target level of force, then begin. When you perform an isometric exercise never hold your breath. Always breathe deeply and naturally, which will be about 10 full breaths in and out at a rate of about 1 second per full breath. Perform each exercise for no less than 7 seconds, and no longer than 10. Try not to rest between each exercise for longer than 10 seconds, which should allow enough time to recover while getting into the next position. Once you have assumed the next isometric exercise angle, perform the exercise in the same way as previously and perform the third angle isometric exercise in the same way. With the triple isometric portion of the exercise completed, try to rest for no longer than 10 seconds before performing the isotonic phase. **NOTE:** If necessary, secure your feet or knees to prevent your lower body from rising as you curl your torso during the exercise. This will help you to focus more on better exercise style and targeting the right muscles.

169

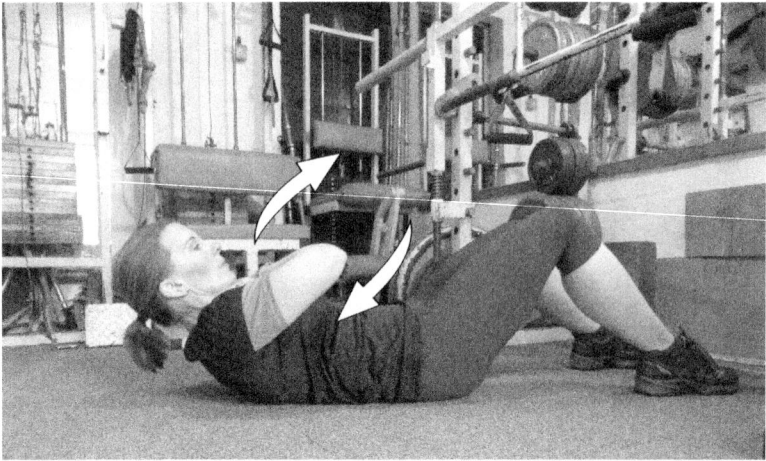
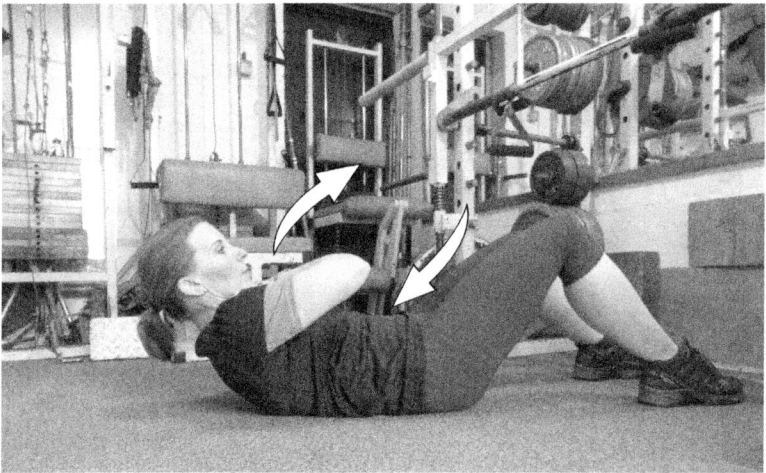
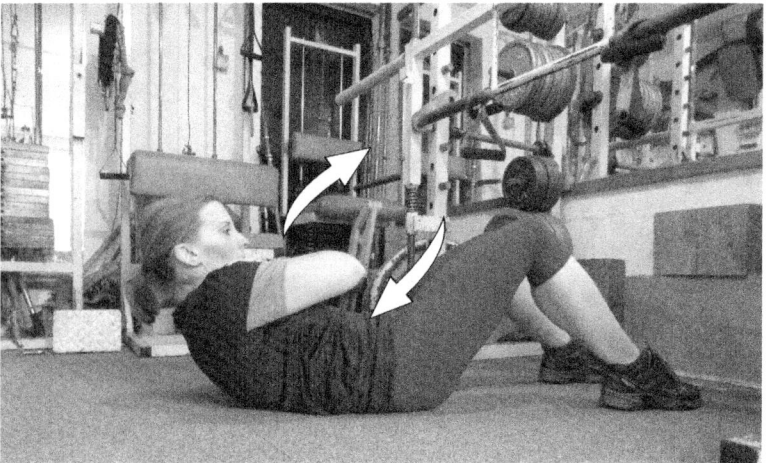

B) Isotonic Bent-Knee Crunch

Maintain the same position as the isometric phase of the exercise, with your back and feet flat on the floor and your knees bent significantly. Place both forearms in front of you resting on your chest and upper abdominals, making two fists with each hand positioned under your chin.

Perform the body curling action in the same way as during the isometric phase. However, you do not stop and hold until you reach the natural top of the movement. At that point, you pause and then slowly return to the starting position to repeat the exercise.

The exercise should be performed in super-slow style with each portion of the exercise (eccentric and concentric) taking between 10 and 12 seconds to complete. This makes it extremely challenging by any standards.

Never hold your breath, and a suggested method of breathing during super-slow repetitions is to breathe in and out one full breath for each second of elapsed time.

Aim to perform one set of three repetitions, but do not be surprised if you can only manage one repetition at super-slow speed.

If this is your limit, even only one repetition performed at super-slow speed will deliver all the results you desire.

Do not sacrifice good exercise style and true super-slow speed in exchange for a greater number of repetitions at a faster speed.

You will gradually increase the number of repetitions you can perform by following the science and adhering to a strict exercise style and good technique.

NOTE: If necessary, secure your feet or knees to prevent your lower body from rising off the floor as you curl your torso. This will help you to focus more on better exercise style and targeting the right muscles.

8. Back Lower – (Triple Position Hold)
A) Isometric Bent Leg Deadlift (Rope / Iso-Bow® / etc.)

First, decide each of the angles you will assume when performing the three successive isometric exercises. Then decide if you will use any equipment or not, and if so, what it will be. If you are going to use any equipment then deploy and test it in advance of beginning both the isometric and isotonic exercise phases for this body part, even if it will only be used for just one of the phases.

We will assume that you will use a rope for the description. Stand with your feet roughly shoulder-width apart and place a length of sturdy rope under both feet. Make sure that the rope is right in the middle of your feet under your arches to help ensure the rope will not slip. Bend and squat slightly down from your knees and hips, keeping your back straight. Take a firm grip on the rope and if needed loop it around your hands. In this position, prepare to use your lower back muscles and glutes as the primary drivers to lift into a deadlift position to perform the exercise. Once you are in the first isometric exercise position, hold at that point. Gradually apply pressure using Dynamic Flexation™ until you have applied the approximate desired target level of intensity. Then begin the first isometric exercise.

When you perform an isometric exercise never hold your breath. Always breathe deeply and naturally, which will be about 10 full breaths in and out at a rate of about 1 second per full breath. Perform each exercise for no less than 7 seconds, and no longer than 10. Try not to rest between each exercise for longer than 10 seconds, which should allow enough time to recover while getting into the next position. Once you have assumed the next isometric exercise angle, perform the exercise in the same way as the previous one, and then perform the third angle isometric exercise in the same way. With the triple isometric portion of the exercise completed, try to rest for no longer than 10 seconds before performing the isotonic phase.

173

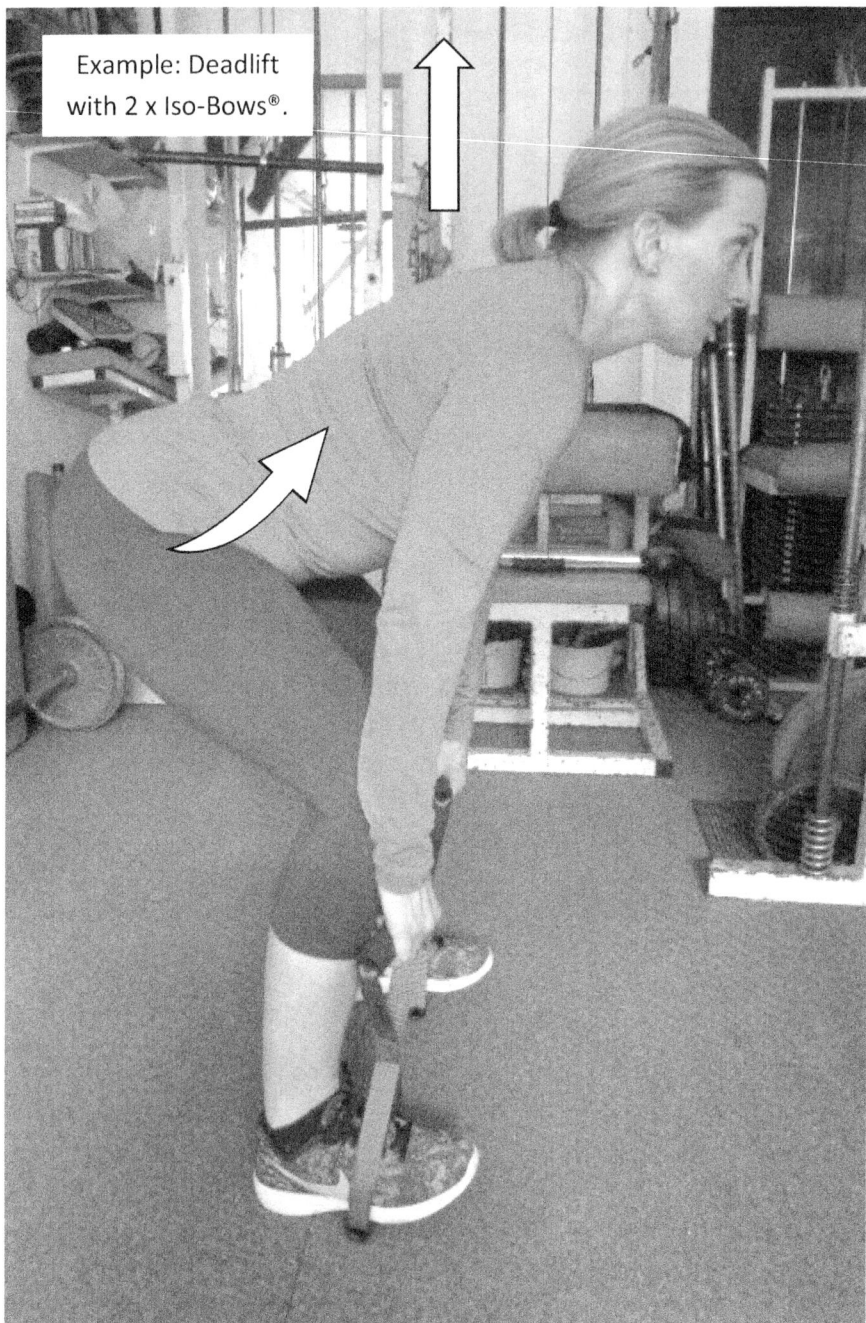

Example: Deadlift with 2 x Iso-Bows®.

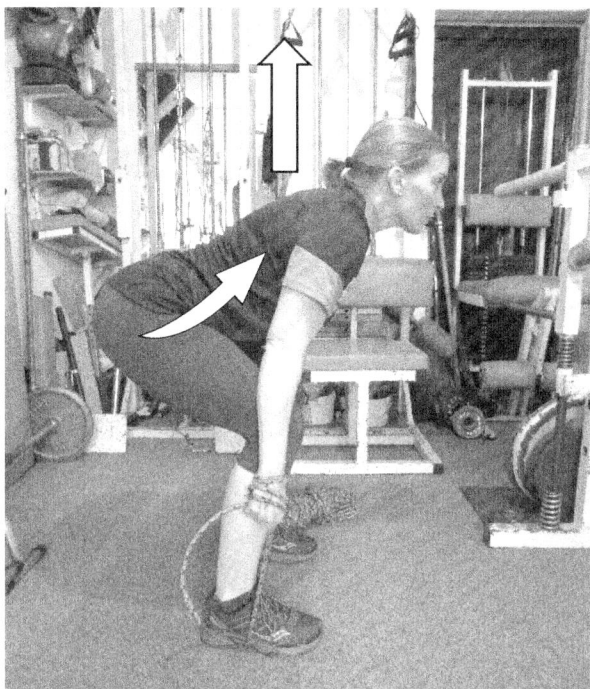

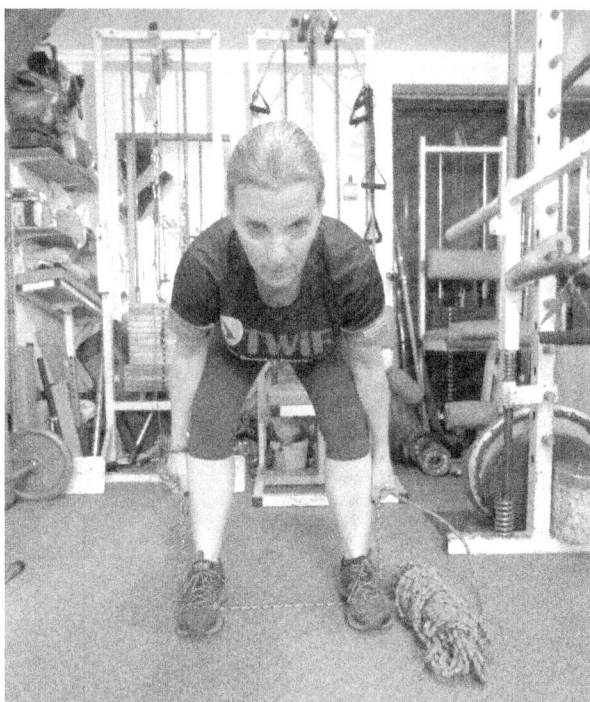

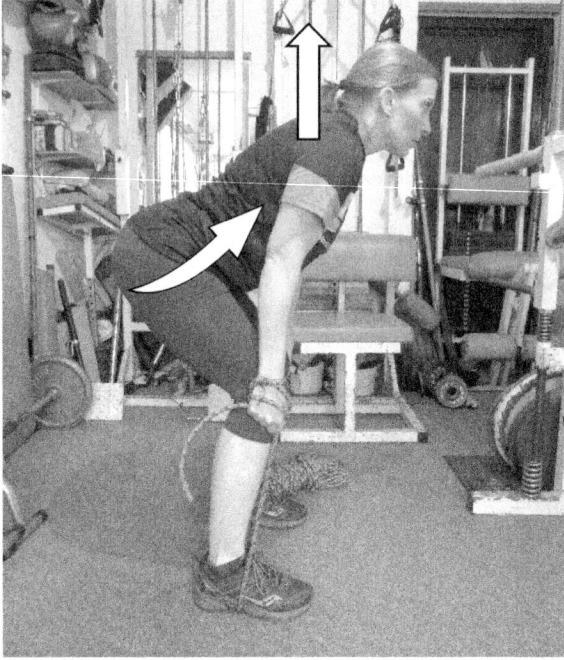

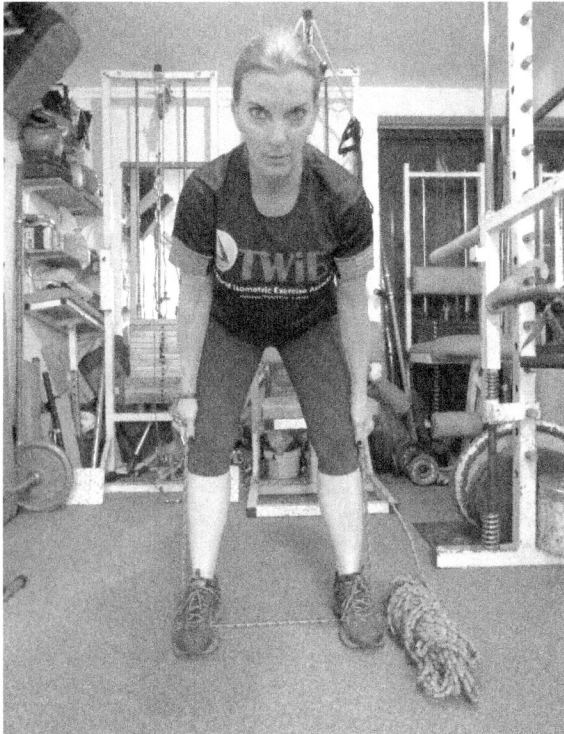

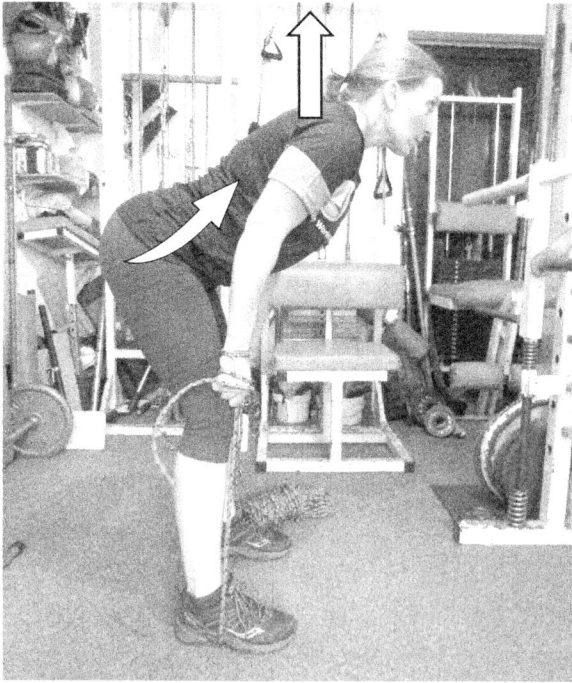

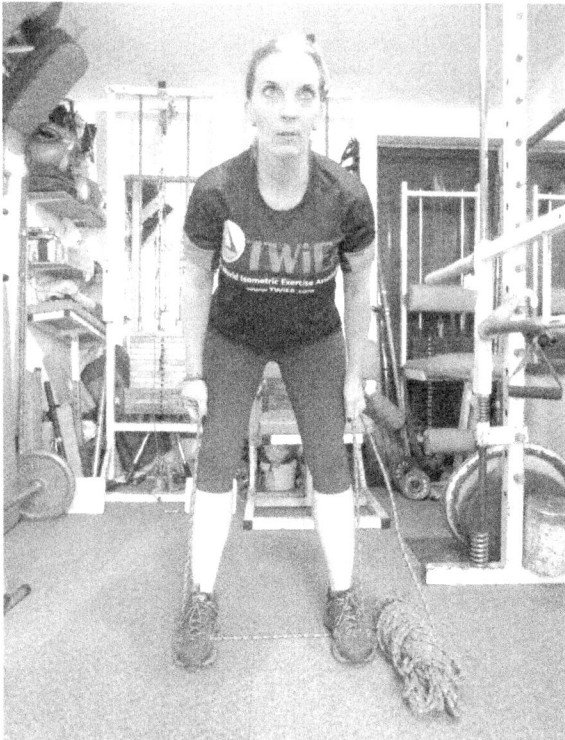

B) Isotonic Floor Hyperextensions

Maintain the same position as the isometric phase of the exercise, lying face down flat out on a floor or mat and with your elbows close to the body. Raise the torso while keeping the legs flat on the floor engaging the lower back muscles as you do so until you reach the highest point of the movement, pause, and then return to the starting position.

The exercise should be performed in super-slow style with each portion of the exercise (eccentric and concentric) taking between 10 and 12 seconds to complete. This makes it extremely challenging by any standards. Never hold your breath, and a suggested method of breathing during super-slow repetitions is to breathe in and out one full breath for each second of elapsed time.

Aim to perform one set of between three repetitions, but do not be surprised if you can only manage one repetition at super-slow speed. If this is your limit, even only one repetition performed at super-slow speed will deliver all the results you desire. Do not sacrifice good exercise style and true super-slow speed in exchange for a greater number of repetitions at a faster speed. You will gradually increase the number of repetitions you can perform by following the science and adhering to a strict exercise style and good technique.

NOTE: The hyperextension exercise is always more effective and focussed on the lower back muscles if the hips and thighs are raised from the floor in a secure position. Ideally, using a dedicated hyperextension bench is always best. However, this can be improvised at home by using a solid footstool (or similar) of enough height. You can use cushions or pillows placed on the footstool to lie on to increase the comfort level. Similarly, if no dedicated bench or footstool is available several think pillows can always be used on the floor to increase the height of the hips and thighs. If raising the height of the hips and thighs, your feet should be secured to prevent them from rising from the floor during the exercise. Using a sofa, heavy chair or bed generally works well enough.

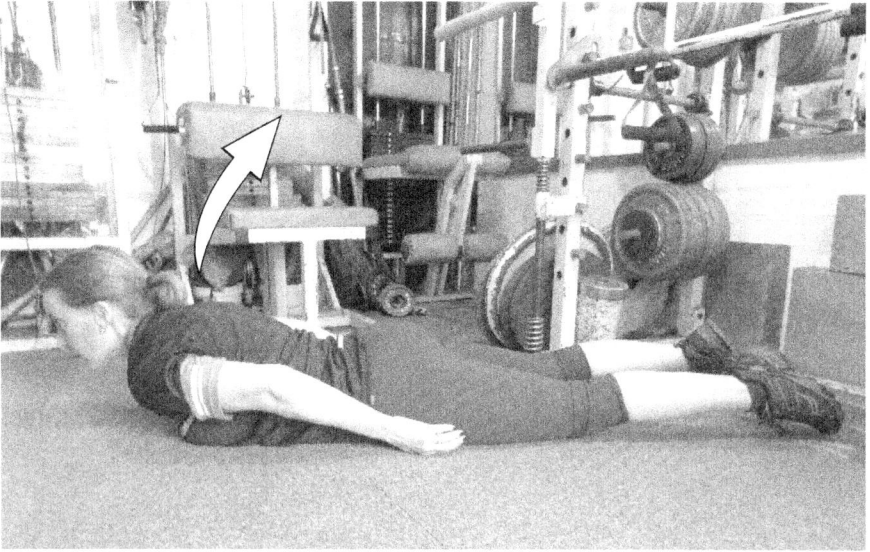

There is only limited ROM (Range Of Motion) involved when performing the floor hyperextension so even though on initial inspection each picture may look the same, it is not. In each picture, the torso has risen ever so slightly higher than in the previous one.

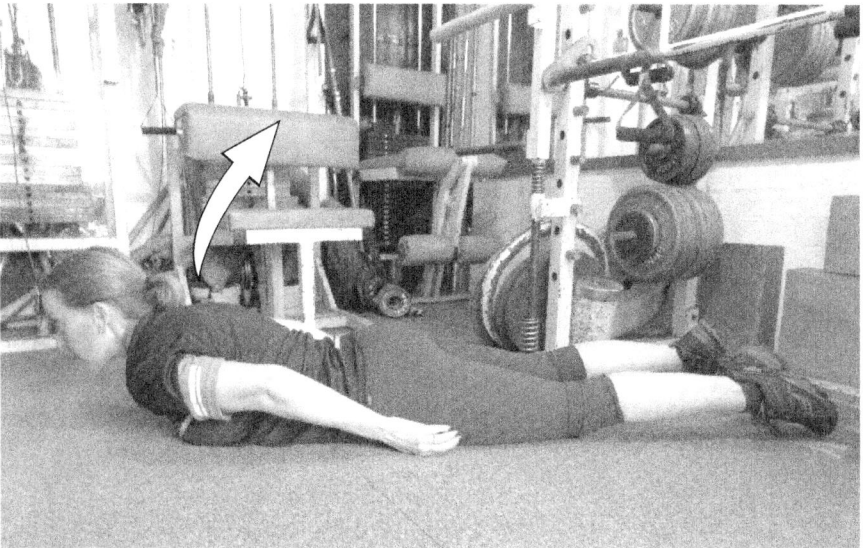

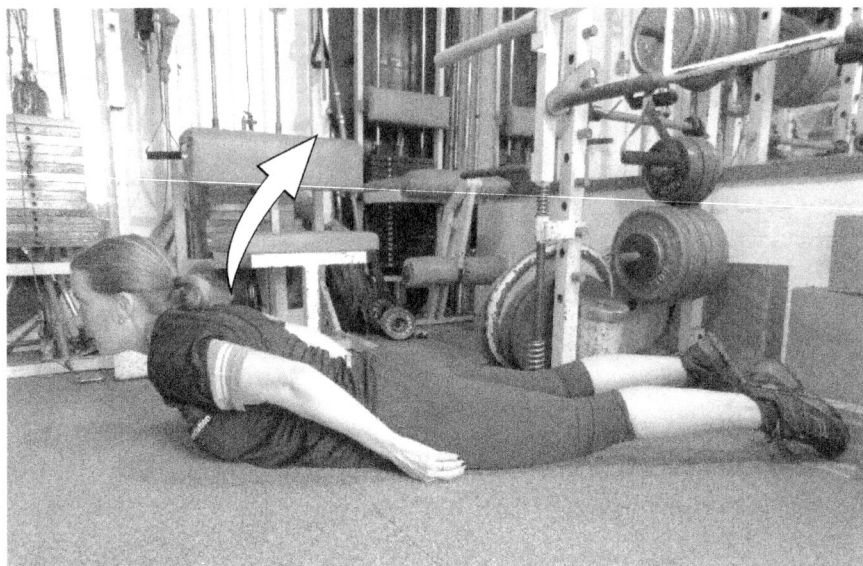

A more effective alternative to floor hyperextensions is the hyperextension on a footstool with the feet secured under something solid at the right height such as a doorway pull-up bar or similar.

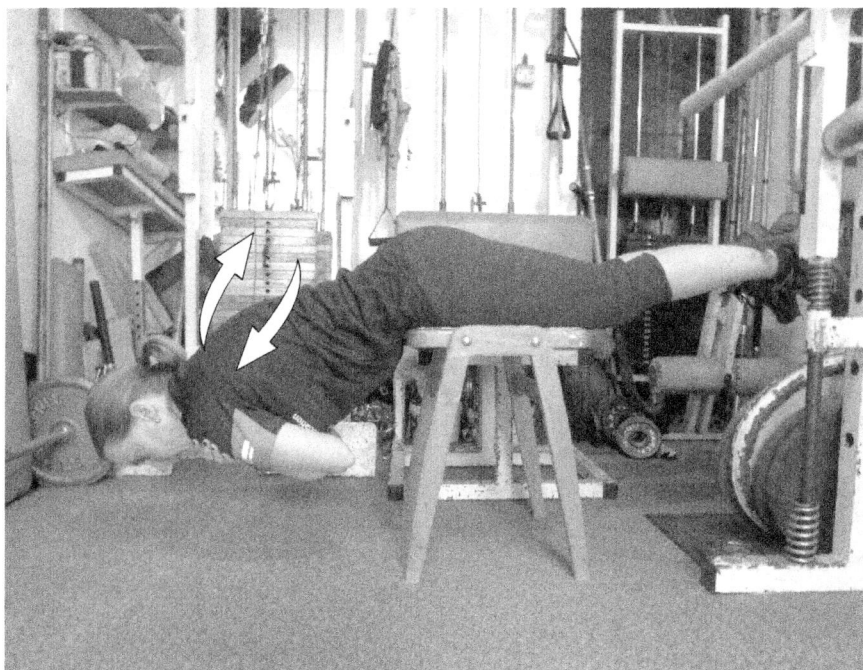

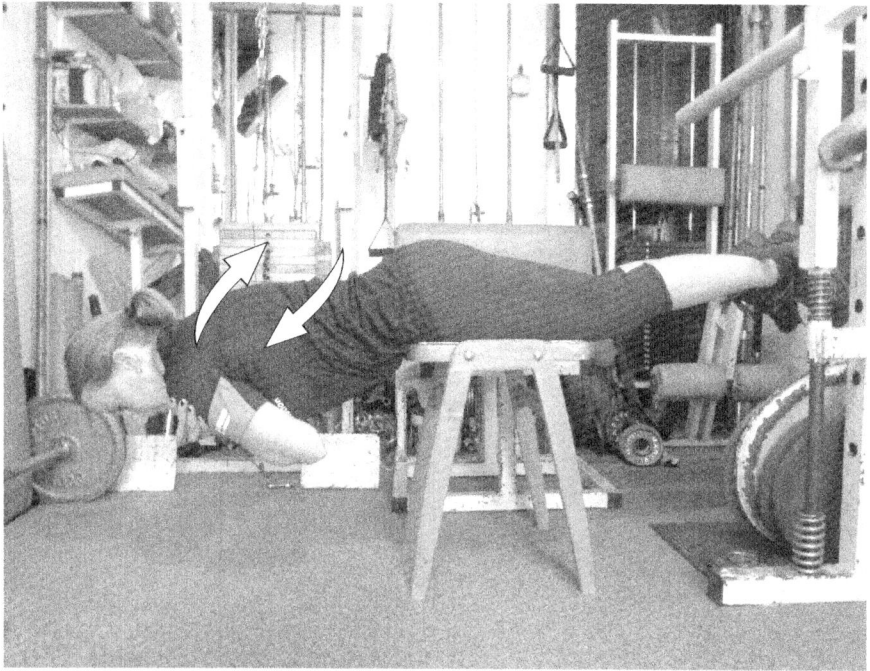

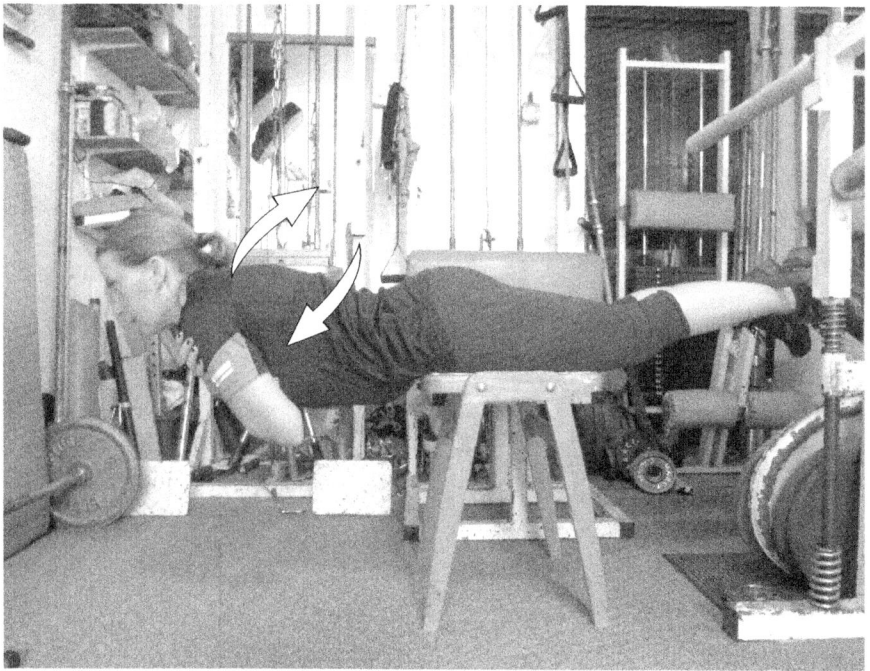

9.   Forearms - Water Bottle Grip (Single, Double or Triple Position Hold)

Ideally, you will need three pairs of plastic water bottles, each with a screw cap, making six bottles in total. Make certain that each pair of bottles is identical in size.

The smallest size bottle should allow you to almost get your fingers wrapped completely around it, the middle size bottle should be big enough to get your fingers partially around, and the largest size should make it challenging to get your fingers wrapped around it.

Fill the bottles to the brim with plain tap water and ensure if possible that there is no air gap. Since water cannot be compressed, it will perfectly counterbalance even the strongest grip that is applied.

Start with the smallest bottle size and work your way up with each set of exercises. Stand upright and hold one bottle in each hand, with your hands and arms slightly away from the body. In this position, apply as much force with your grip as you try to compress and crush the bottle.

The harder you engage the muscles, the more intense the exercise becomes, so always be sure to exercise at an intensity that best suits your current ability. When you perform an isometric exercise never hold your breath.

Always breathe deeply and naturally, which will be about 10 full breaths in and out at a rate of about 1 second per full breath. Perform each exercise for no less than 7 seconds, and no longer than 10.

NOTE: Do not use a glass bottle, a can, or a plastic bottle filled with carbonated liquid as any of these may burst or shatter.

We choose to only use one large bottle because of the weight of it when filled with liquid. The bottle can be used to exercise each hand individually, or if it is big enough and/or your hands are small enough, then both hands at the same time.

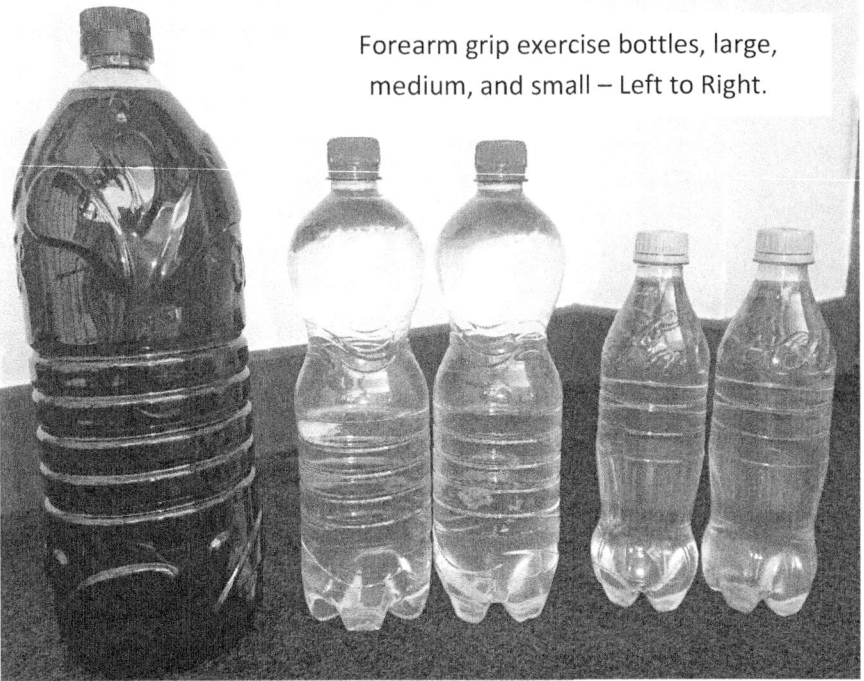

Forearm grip exercise bottles, large, medium, and small – Left to Right.

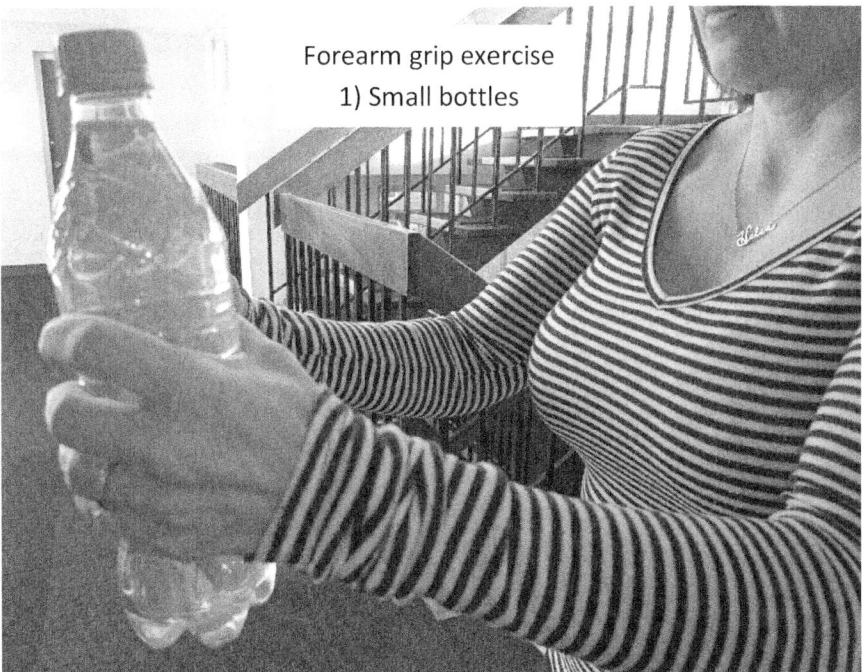

Forearm grip exercise
1) Small bottles

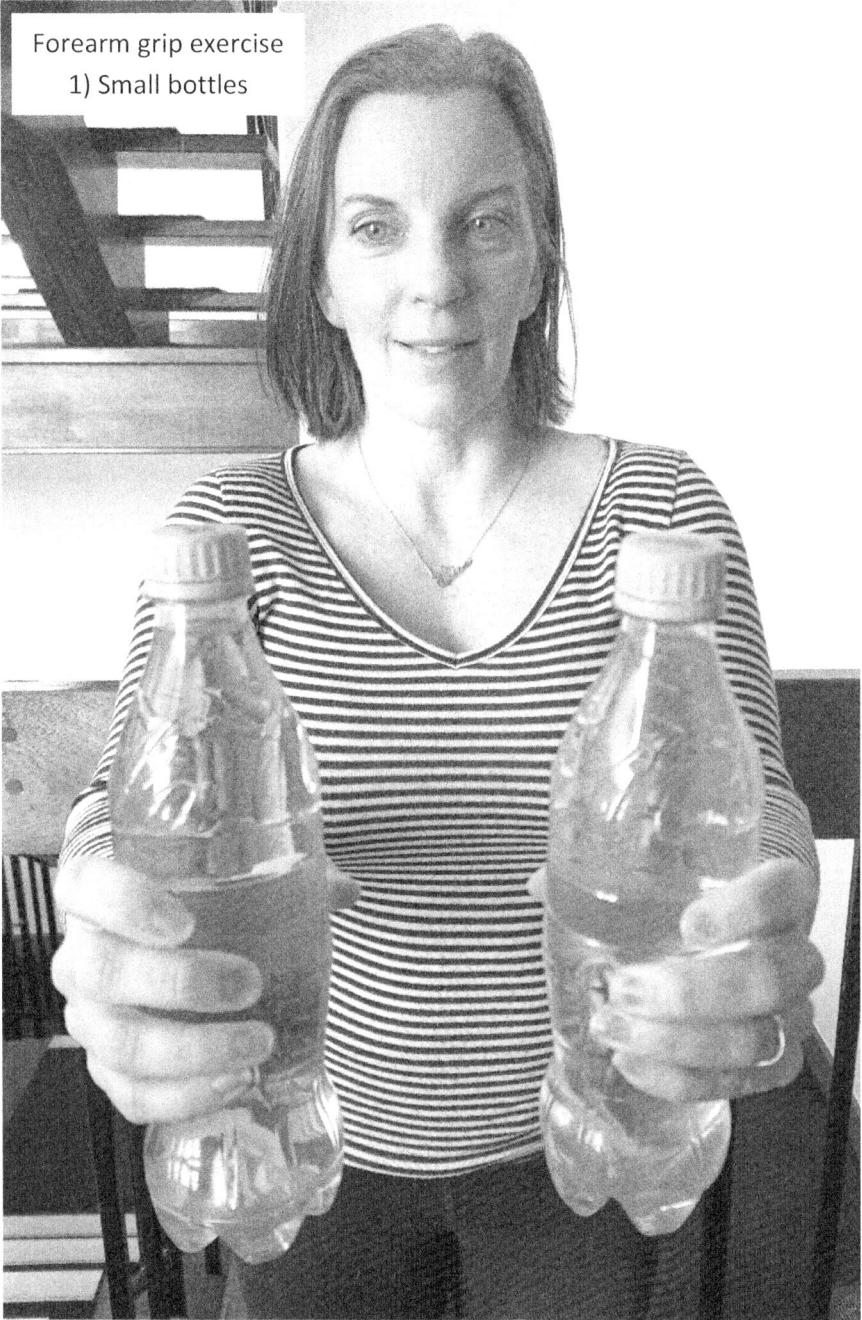

Forearm grip exercise
1) Small bottles

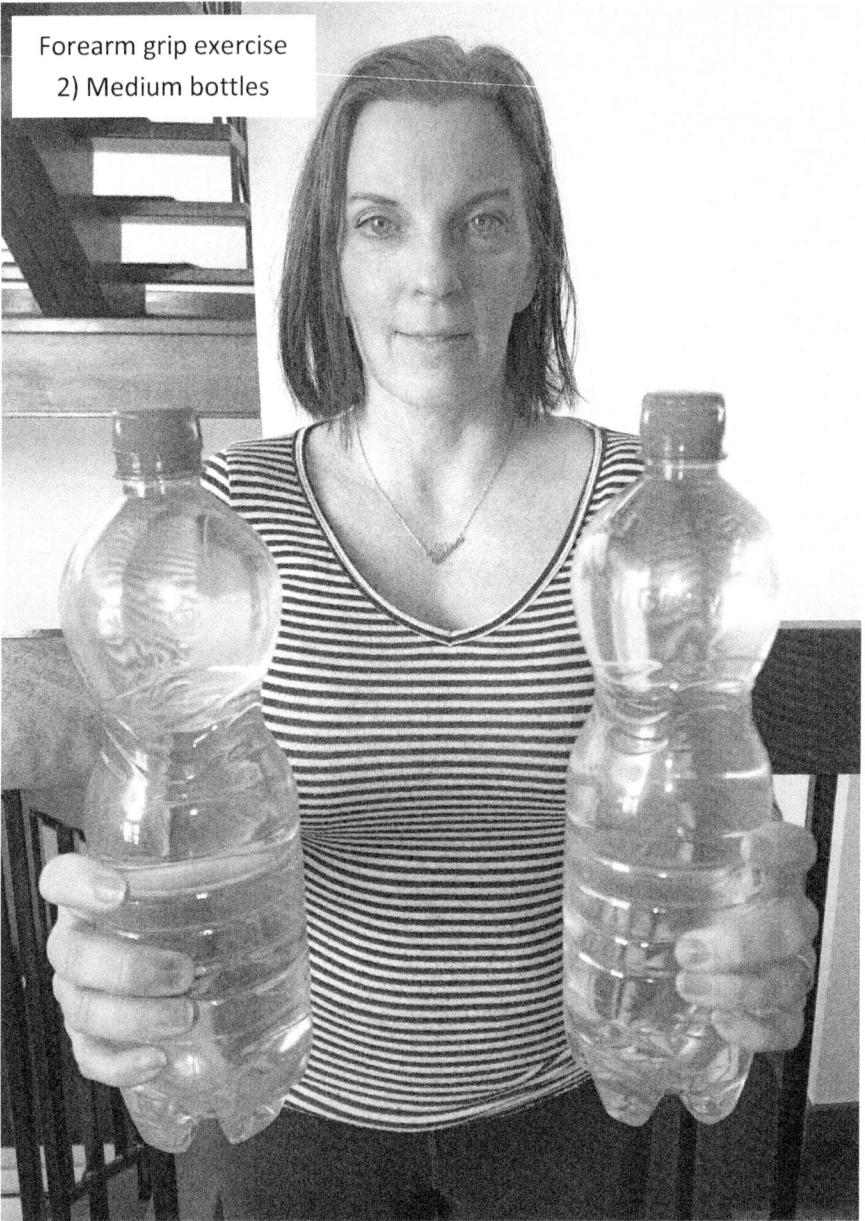

Forearm grip exercise
2) Medium bottles

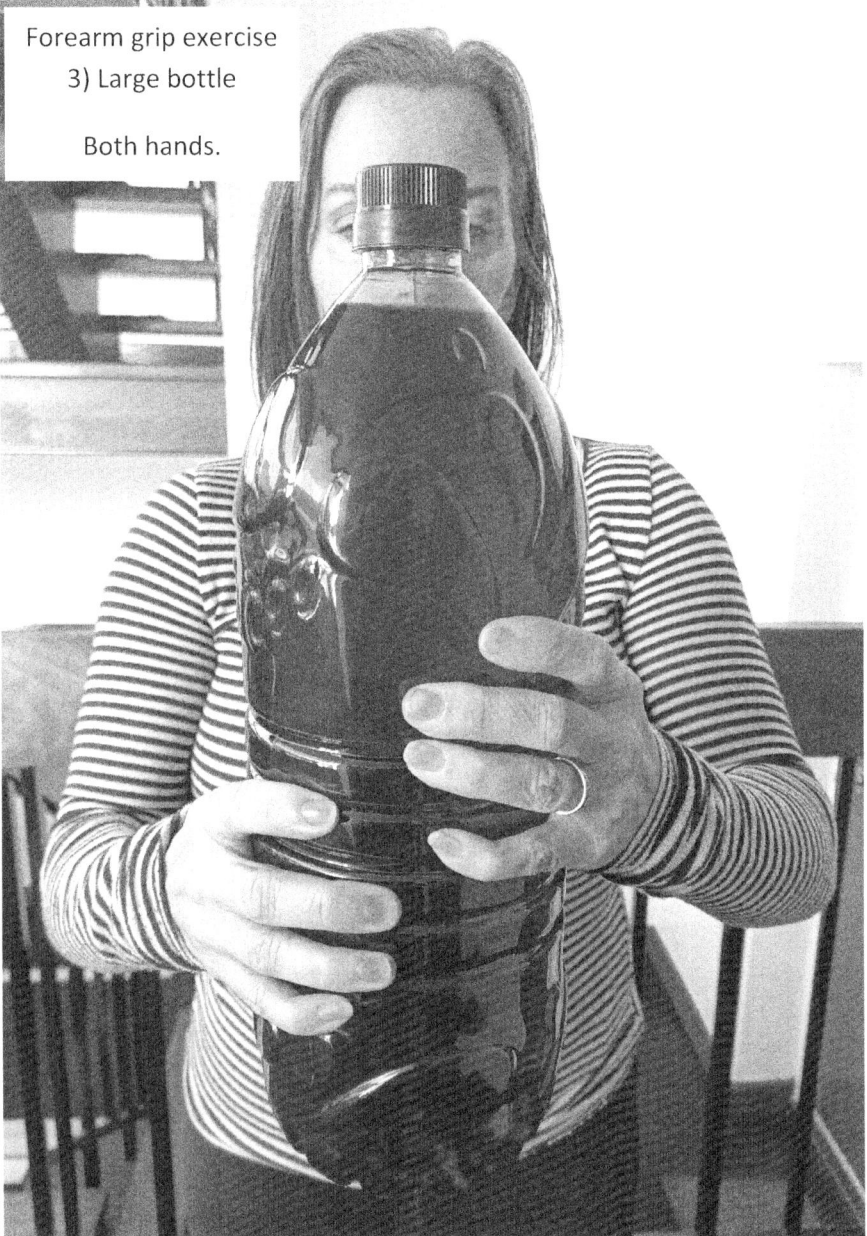

Forearm grip exercise
3) Large bottle

Both hands.

10.   Back – Upper - (Rope / Iso-Bow® / Hands etc.)
A) Isometric Chest-Level Pull-Apart (Triple Position)

First, decide each of the angles you will assume when performing the three successive isometric exercises. Then decide if you will use any equipment or not, and if so, what it will be. If you are going to use any equipment then deploy and test it in advance of beginning both the isometric and isotonic exercise phases for this body part, even if it will only be used for just one of the phases.

Stand upright and raise your arms to upper chest level with elbows bent out sideways until they are roughly parallel to the floor. Inter-hook your fingers together or use any other solid grip that will not slip. If you are using rope or a towel, then make sure you grip it securely. You can loop the rope around hour hands if needed. An Iso-Bow® or similar will provide you with the best grip.

Attempt to pull your hands apart and position them in the correct position for the first isometric exercise. Your grip prevents your hands from being pulled apart as you engage the upper back, shoulder, and neck muscles. Gradually apply pressure using Dynamic Flexation™ until you have applied the approximate desired target level of intensity, then begin the first isometric exercise.

When you perform an isometric exercise never hold your breath. Always breathe deeply and naturally, which will be about 10 full breaths in and out at a rate of about 1 second per full breath. Perform each exercise for no less than 7 seconds, and no longer than 10. Try not to rest between each exercise for longer than 10 seconds, which should allow enough time to recover while getting into the next position.

Once you have assumed the next isometric exercise angle, perform the exercise in the same way as the previous one, and then perform the third angle isometric exercise in the same way. With the triple isometric portion of the exercise completed, try to rest for no longer than 10 seconds before performing the isotonic phase.

189

Triple Position Isometric Exercise

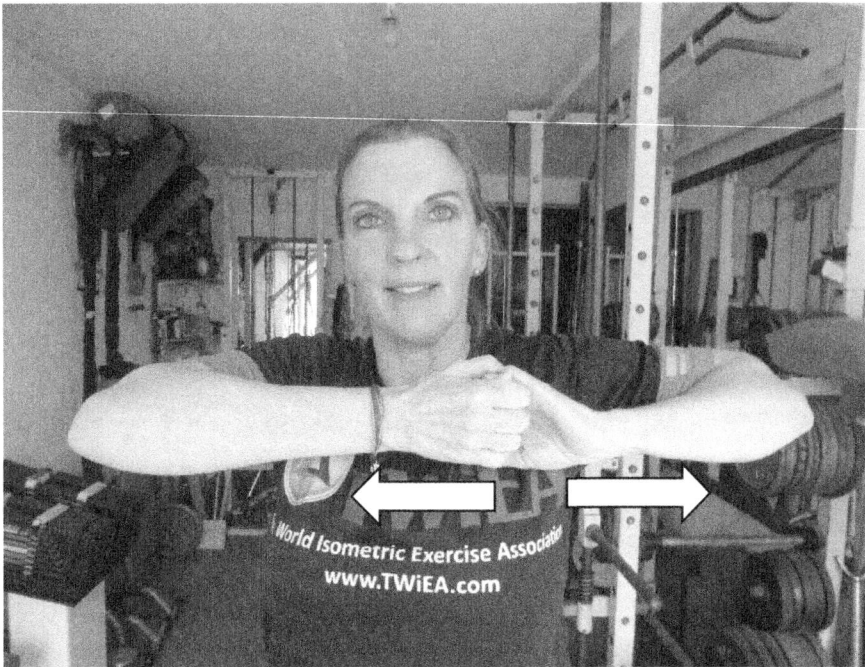

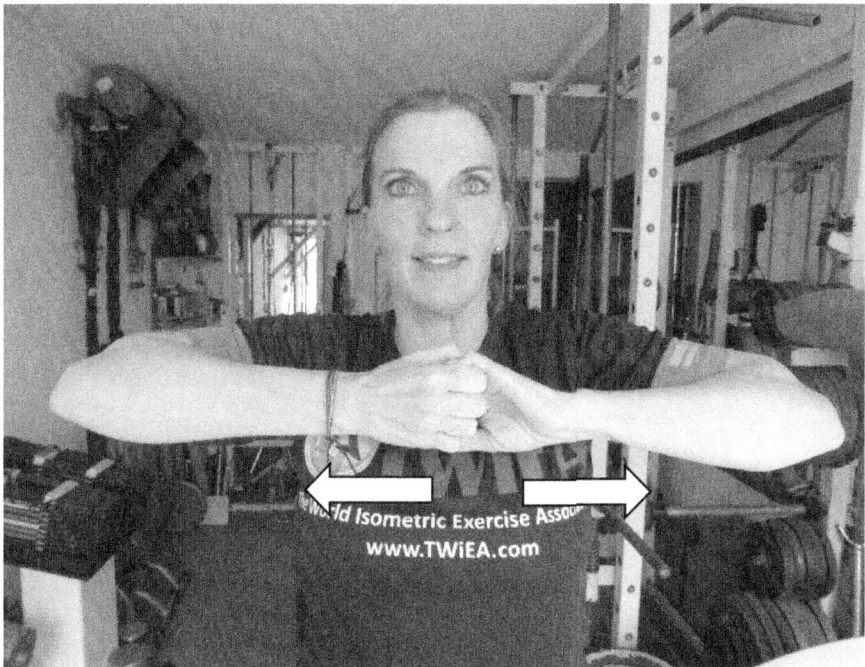

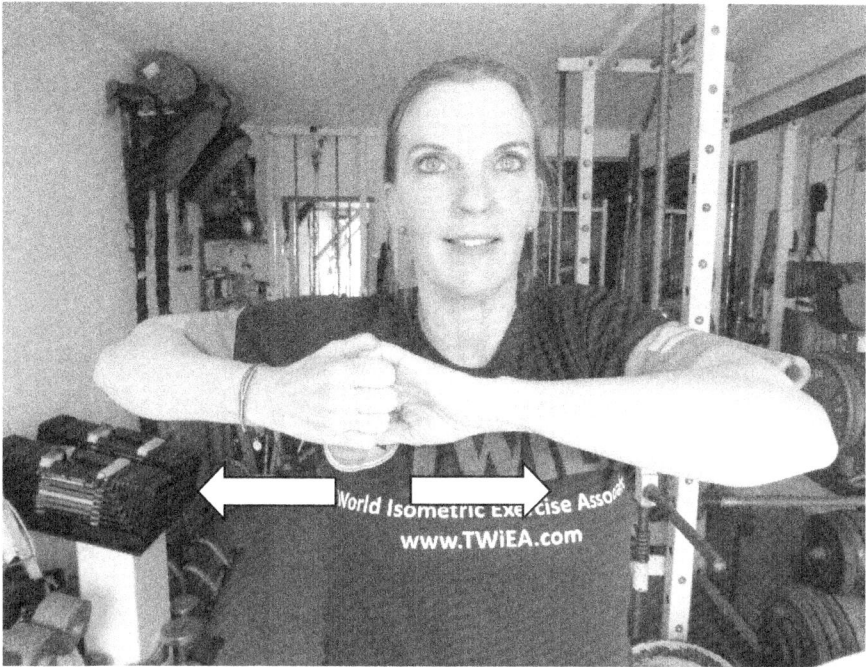

B) Upper Back Isotonic Exercise - Iso-Bow® Seated Knee Row

Sit upright on a solid object such as a chair, car seat or bench, bending forwards only from the hips, and always keep your back straight. Lift one knee and comfortably wrap the Iso-Bow® around in front of it, or a towel or with your hands, pull back with the handles as you engage your upper back muscles, keeping your elbows close to your body as you do so. The exercise should be performed in super-slow style with each portion of the exercise (eccentric and concentric) taking between 10 and 12 seconds to complete. This makes it extremely challenging by any standards. Never hold your breath, and a suggested method of breathing during super-slow repetitions is to breathe in and out one full breath for each second of elapsed time. Aim to perform one set of three repetitions, but do not be surprised if you can only manage one repetition at super-slow speed. If this is your limit, even only one or two repetitions performed at super-slow speed will deliver all the results you desire. Do not sacrifice good exercise style and true super-slow speed in exchange for a greater number of repetitions at a faster speed. You will gradually increase the number of repetitions you can perform by following the science and adhering to a strict exercise style and good technique.

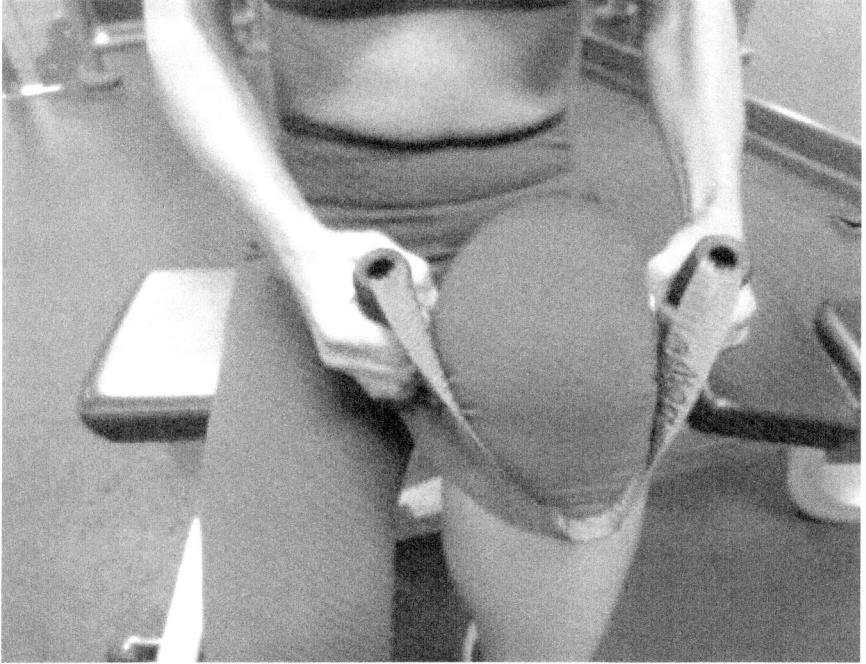

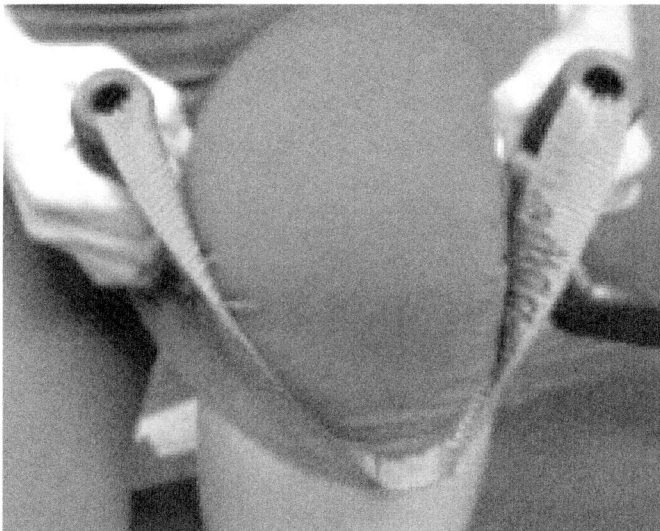

NOTE: Instead of using an Iso-Bow® you can wrap your hands around your knee and interlock your fingers.

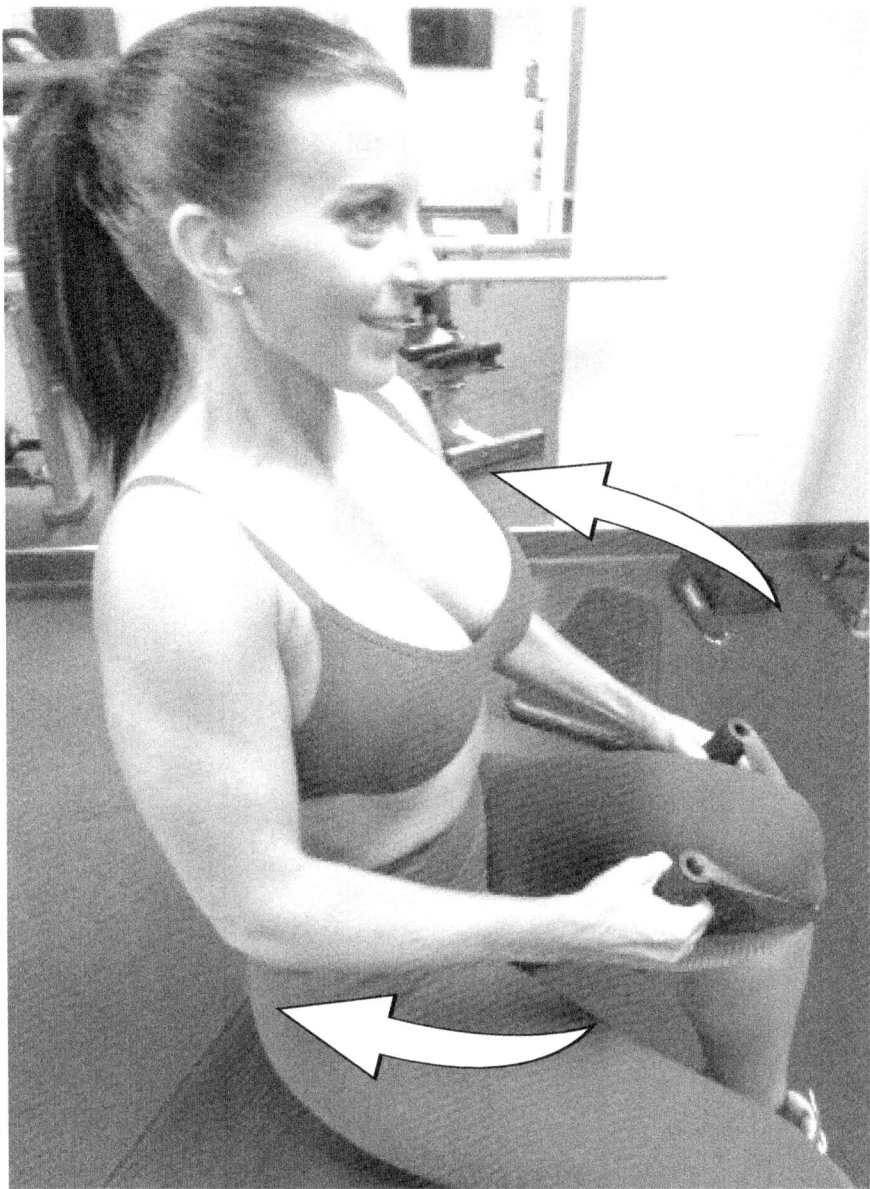

The Muscle-up For Menopause™ (MUM™) Course – 2nd Month at a Glance

1. Legs - Upper
    a. Isometric
        i. Split Squat (Triple Position Hold) (Left Leg) (Rear Foot Elevated on Bench / Chair / Footstool)
    b. Isotonic
        i. Split Squats (Left and Right Leg) (Rear Foot Elevated on Bench / Chair / Footstool)
2. Legs - Upper
    a. Isometric
        i. Split Squat (Triple Position Hold) (Right Leg) (Rear Foot Elevated on Bench / Chair / Footstool)
    b. Isotonic
        i. Split Squats (Left and Right Leg) (Rear Foot Elevated on Bench / Chair / Footstool)
3. Legs - Calf's
    a. Isometric
        i. Isometric Calf Double Leg Wall Push (Triple Position Hold)
    b. Isotonic
        i. Isotonic Double Heel Raise
4. Triceps
    a. Isometric
        i. Triceps Push Down (Rope / Iso-Gym® / Towel / Doorway Pull-Up Bar / Door) (Triple Position Hold)
    b. Isotonic
        i. Triceps 20 to 40 Degree Front Press (Table / Wall / Doorway Pull-up Bar etc.)
5. Biceps
    a. Isometric
        i. Doorway Pull-up Bar Biceps Curl (Mid to High Angle Position) (Triple Position Hold) (Grip Either Bar or 2 Looped Iso-Bows®)
    b. Isotonic

        i. Doorway Pull-up Bar Biceps Curl (Mid to High Angle Position) (Grip Either Bar or 2 Looped Iso-Bows®)

6. Abdominals
   a. Isometric
      i. Abdominal set 1
         1. Isometric Bent-Knee Trunk Crunch (Triple Position Hold) (Hands/Arms Resisted)
         2. Isotonic Bent-Knee Crunch (Hands/Arms Resisted)
7. Abdominals
      i. Abdominal set 2
         1. Isometric Kneeling Side Bend (Iso-Bow® Loop Secured Under Each Knee / Rope or Towel under both)
         2. Isotonic Kneeling Side Bend (Iso-Bow® Loop Secured Under Each Knee / Rope or Towel under both)
8. Back - Upper
   a. Isometric
      i. Latissimus Overhead Pull-Apart (Rope / Iso-Bow® / Towel / Hands) (Triple Position Hold)
   b. Isotonic
      i. Seated Pull-ups (Doorway Pull-up Bar)
9. Shoulders
   a. Isometric
      i. Front Raise (Left Side) (Rope / Iso-Bow® / Towel / Hand) (Triple Position Hold)
   b. Isotonic
      i. Front Raise (Left Side) (Rope / Iso-Bow® / Towel / Hands)
10. Shoulders
   a. Isometric
      i. Front Raise (Right Side) (Rope / Iso-Bow® / Towel / Hand) (Triple Position Hold)
   b. Isotonic
      i. Front Raise (Right Side) (Rope / Iso-Bow® / Towel / Hands)

1. Legs – Upper
A) Isometric Split Squat (Triple Position Hold) (Left Leg) (Rear Foot Elevated on Bench / Chair / Footstool)

First, decide each of the angles you will assume when performing the three successive isometric exercises. Then decide if you will use any equipment or not, and if so, what it will be. If you are going to use any equipment then deploy and test it in advance of beginning both the isometric and isotonic exercise phases for this body part, even if it will only be used for just one of the phases.

We will assume that you are using no equipment for this exercise. It is important to determine the correct distance you need to stand away from the footstool. This might take a few experimental moves, to begin with. The closer you stand to the footstool then the greater the focus that is placed on the front upper thighs. The ideal position is when you feel a slight stretch in the hip flexor at the lowest point of the exercise when the rear knee touches a folded towel you have preplaced just in front of the footstool.

Stand in front of the towel. Place one leg back so that the top of the foot is positioned on the top of the footstool etc. If you need to use something to touch to aid your balance, then do so. However, it is best to avoid this, if possible, since the object is to activate as many of the core-supporting muscles as possible during the exercise.

Perform the triple isometric phase for one leg immediately followed by the isotonic phase before exercising the other leg in the same way. Keep your body upright and head up as you bend the knee of the front leg to descend into the first isometric exercise position using Dynamic Flexation™ as you engage the target muscles as the primary driving force. Once you have applied the approximate desired target level of intensity, then begin the first isometric exercise.

When you perform an isometric exercise never hold your breath. Always breathe deeply and naturally, which will be about 10 full breaths in and out at a rate of about 1 second per full breath. Perform each exercise for no less than 7 seconds, and no longer than 10. Try not to rest between each exercise for longer than 10 seconds, which should allow enough time to recover while getting into the next position. Once you have assumed the next isometric exercise angle, perform the exercise in the same way as the previous one, and then perform the third angle isometric exercise in the same way. With the triple isometric portion of the exercise completed, try to rest for no longer than 10 seconds before performing the isotonic phase.

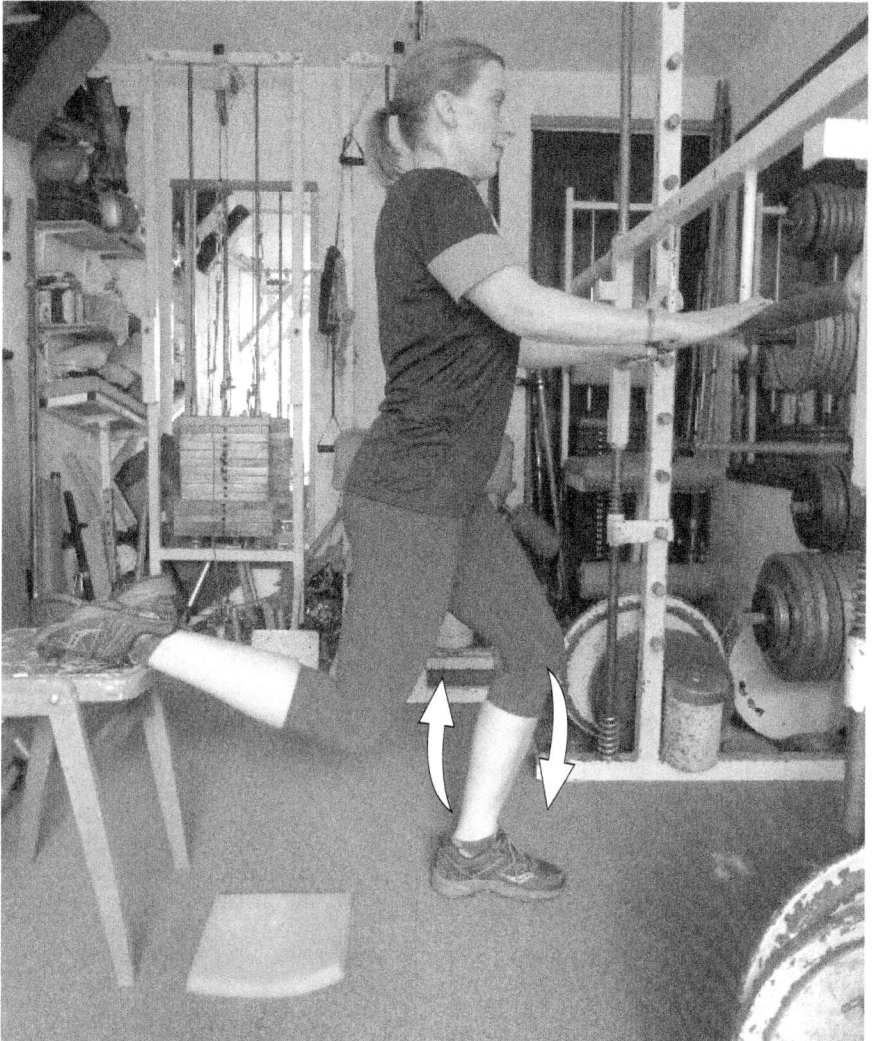

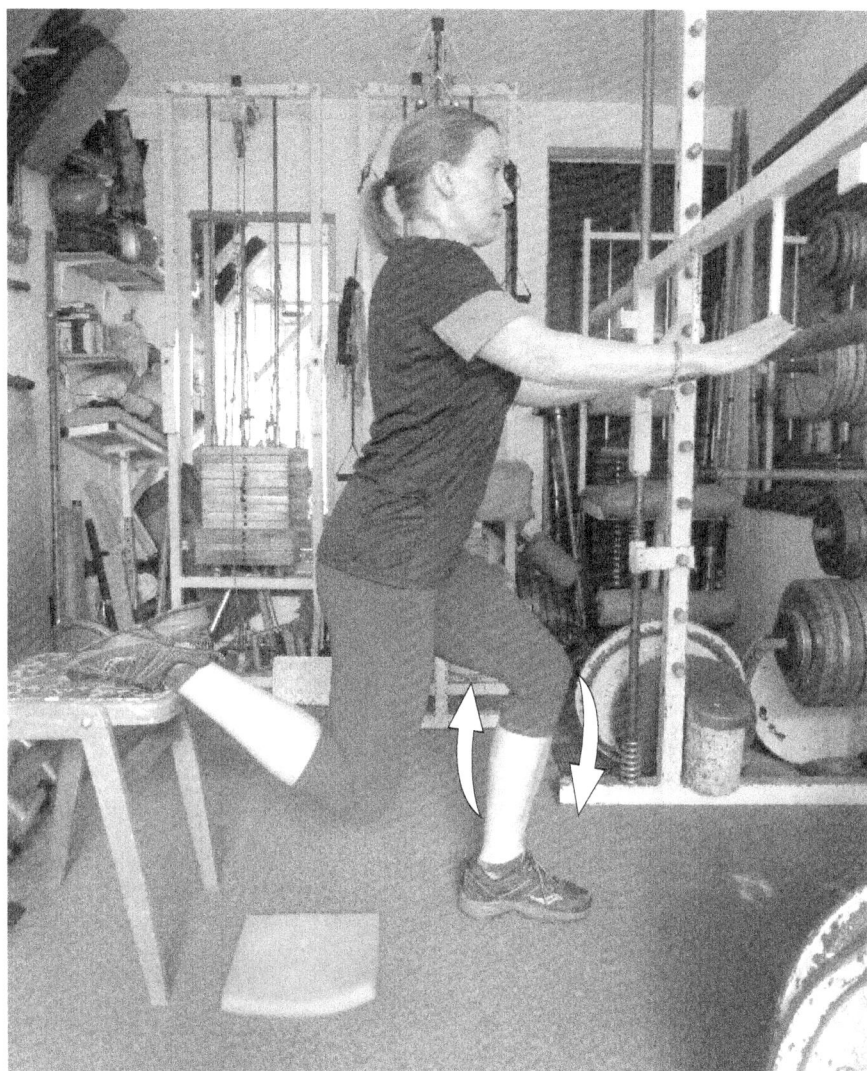

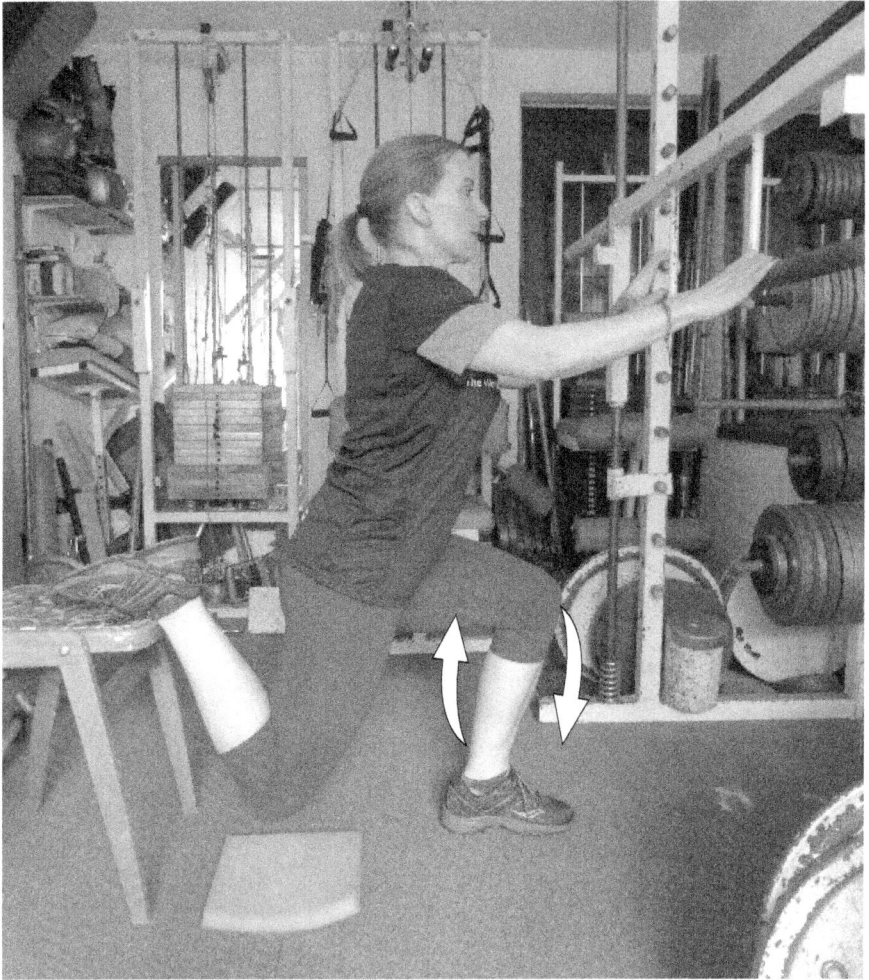

Split squat variation with rope to provide additional resistance during the isometric phase.

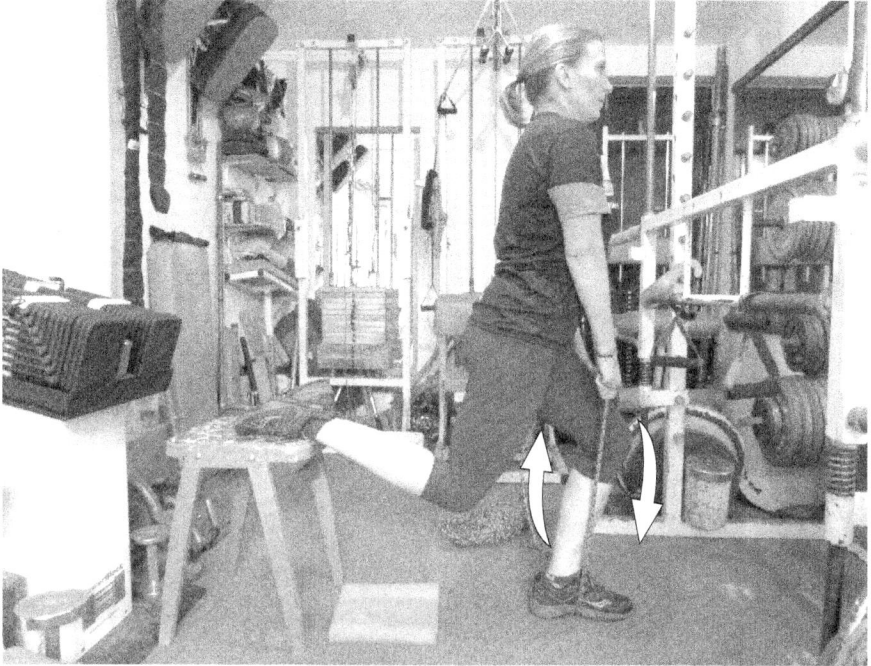

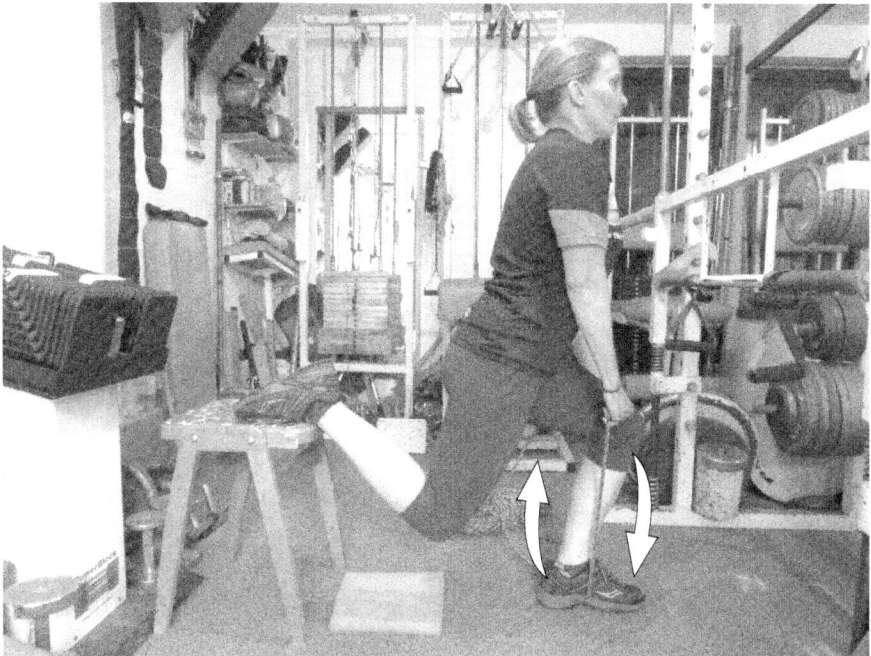

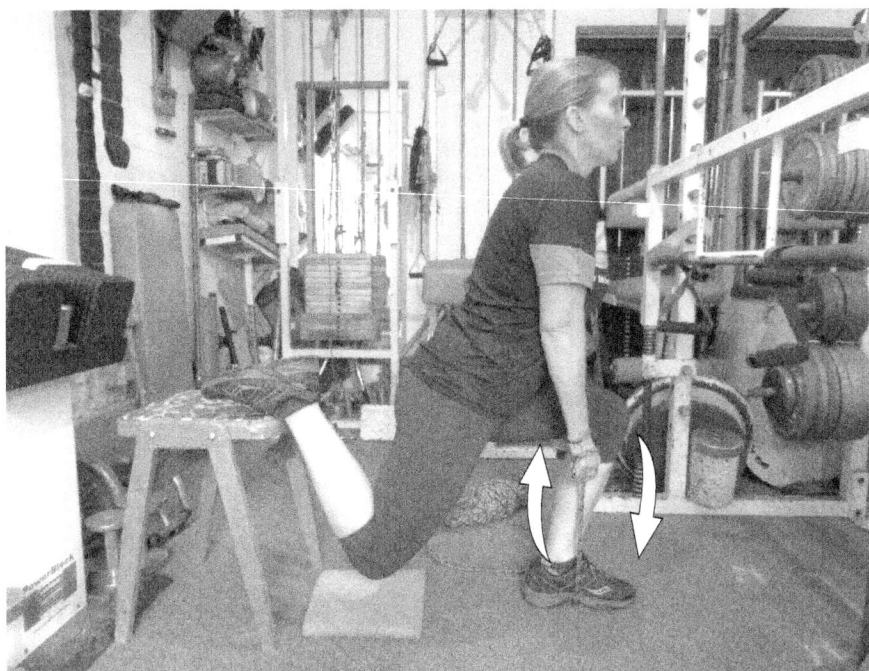

Below and on the next page is the same series of exercise positions as viewed from the front.

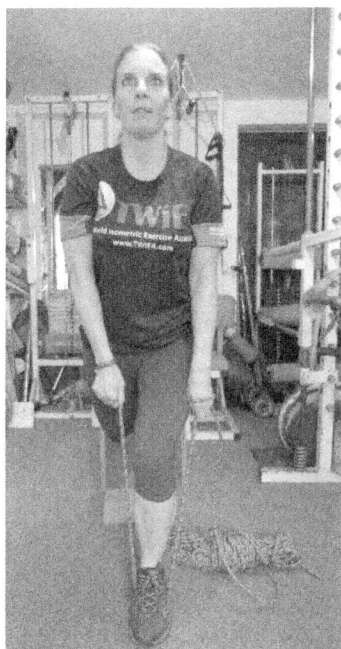

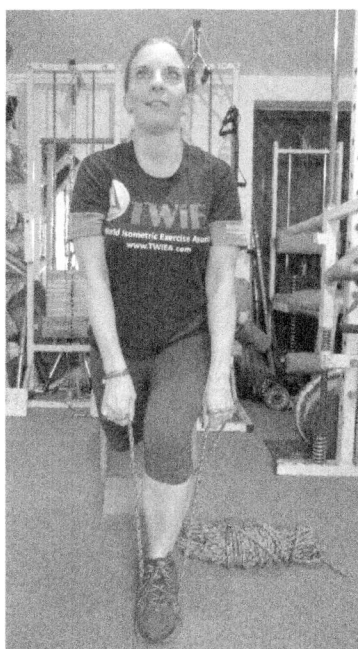

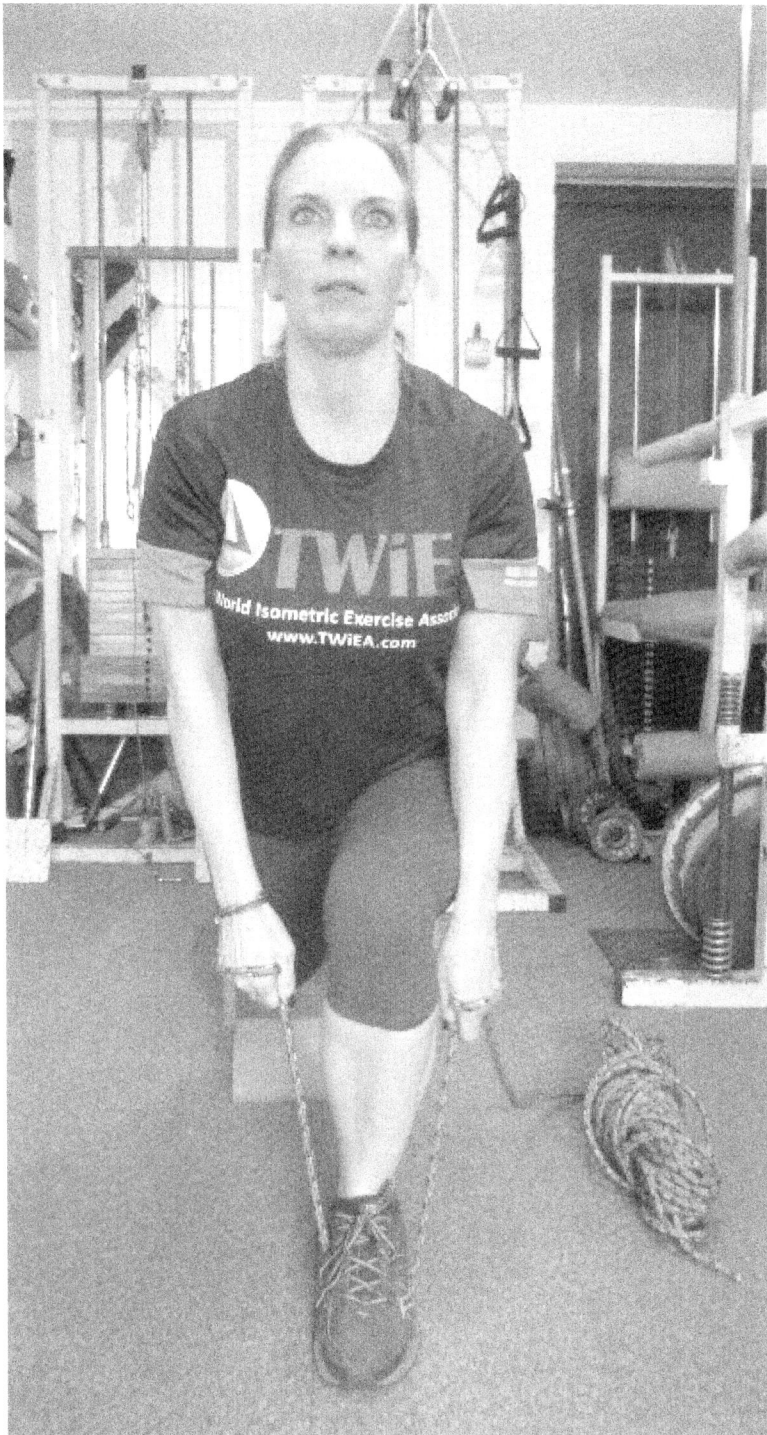

B) Isotonic Split Squats (Left and Right Leg) (Rear Foot Elevated on Bench / Chair / Footstool)

Continuing from the triple position isometric phase, with the feet, knees, arms, and hands in the same positions.

Start in either the upper split squat position and descend to the lowest point of the movement, pause, and then return to the starting position to repeat the exercise.

The exercise should be performed in super-slow style with each portion of the exercise (eccentric and concentric) taking between 10 and 12 seconds to complete.

This makes it extremely challenging by any standards. Never hold your breath, and a suggested method of breathing during super-slow repetitions is to breathe in and out one full breath for each second of elapsed time.

Aim to perform one set of three repetitions, but do not be surprised if you can only manage one repetition at super-slow speed.

If this is your limit, even only one repetition performed at super-slow speed will deliver all the results you desire.

Do not sacrifice good exercise style and true super-slow speed in exchange for a greater number of repetitions at a faster speed.

You will gradually increase the number of repetitions you can perform by following the science and adhering to a strict exercise style and good technique. Please see the picture on the following page.

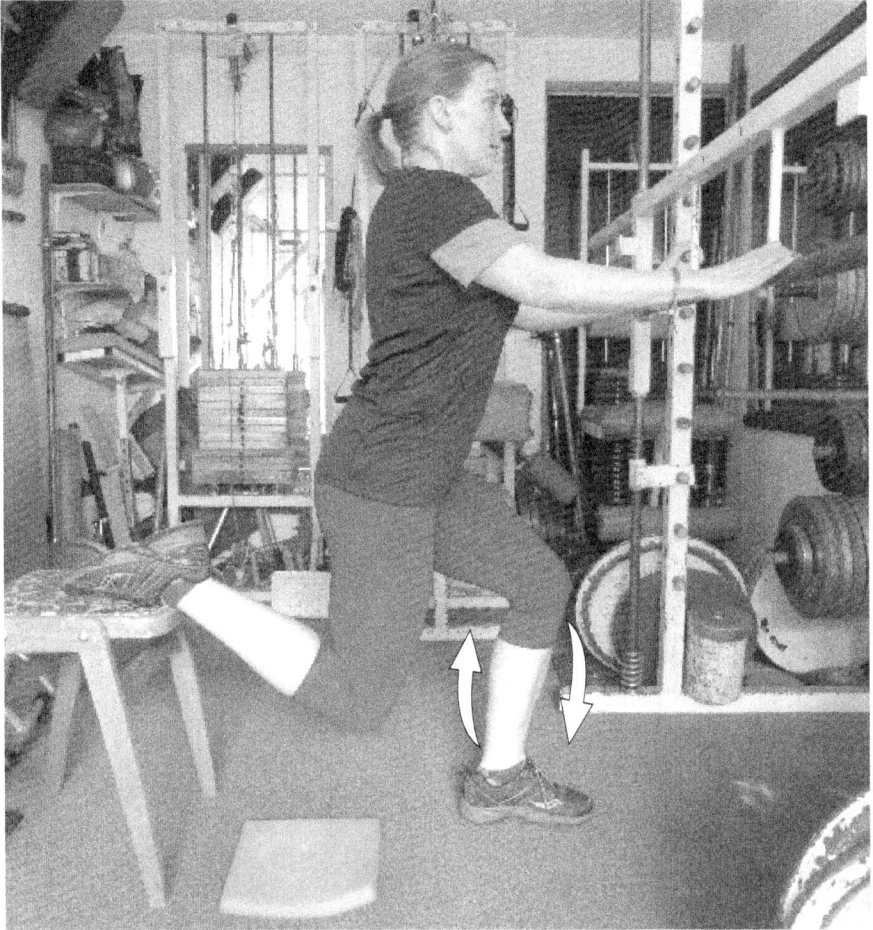

1. Legs - Calf's
A) Isometric Calf Double Leg Wall Push (Triple Position)

First, decide each of the angles you will assume when performing the three successive isometric exercises. There is a limited range of motion in the heel raise exercise so this will require a little thought and preplanning. Then decide if you will use any equipment or not, and if so, what it will be.

If you are going to use any equipment then deploy and test it in advance of beginning both the isometric and isotonic exercise phases for this body part, even if it will only be used for just one of the phases. Face a wall or solid door which closes away from you so it cannot accidentally open or be opened during the exercise. Place your feet roughly shoulder-width apart, with your legs straight and toes facing forwards.

Lean slightly forward towards the wall or door and place both hands flat on the surface at approximately shoulder height as if you intend to push it over. Attempt to raise the heels of each foot to the correct position for the first isometric exercise. Gradually apply pressure using Dynamic Flexation™ until you have applied the approximate desired target level of intensity, then begin the first isometric exercise.

When you perform an isometric exercise never hold your breath. Always breathe deeply and naturally, which will be about 10 full breaths in and out at a rate of about 1 second per full breath. Perform each exercise for no less than 7 seconds, and no longer than 10. Try not to rest between each exercise for longer than 10 seconds, which should allow enough time to recover while getting into the next position.

Once you have assumed the next isometric exercise angle, perform the exercise in the same way as the previous one, and then perform the third angle isometric exercise in the same way.

With the triple isometric portion of the exercise completed, try to rest for no longer than 10 seconds before performing the isotonic phase.

207

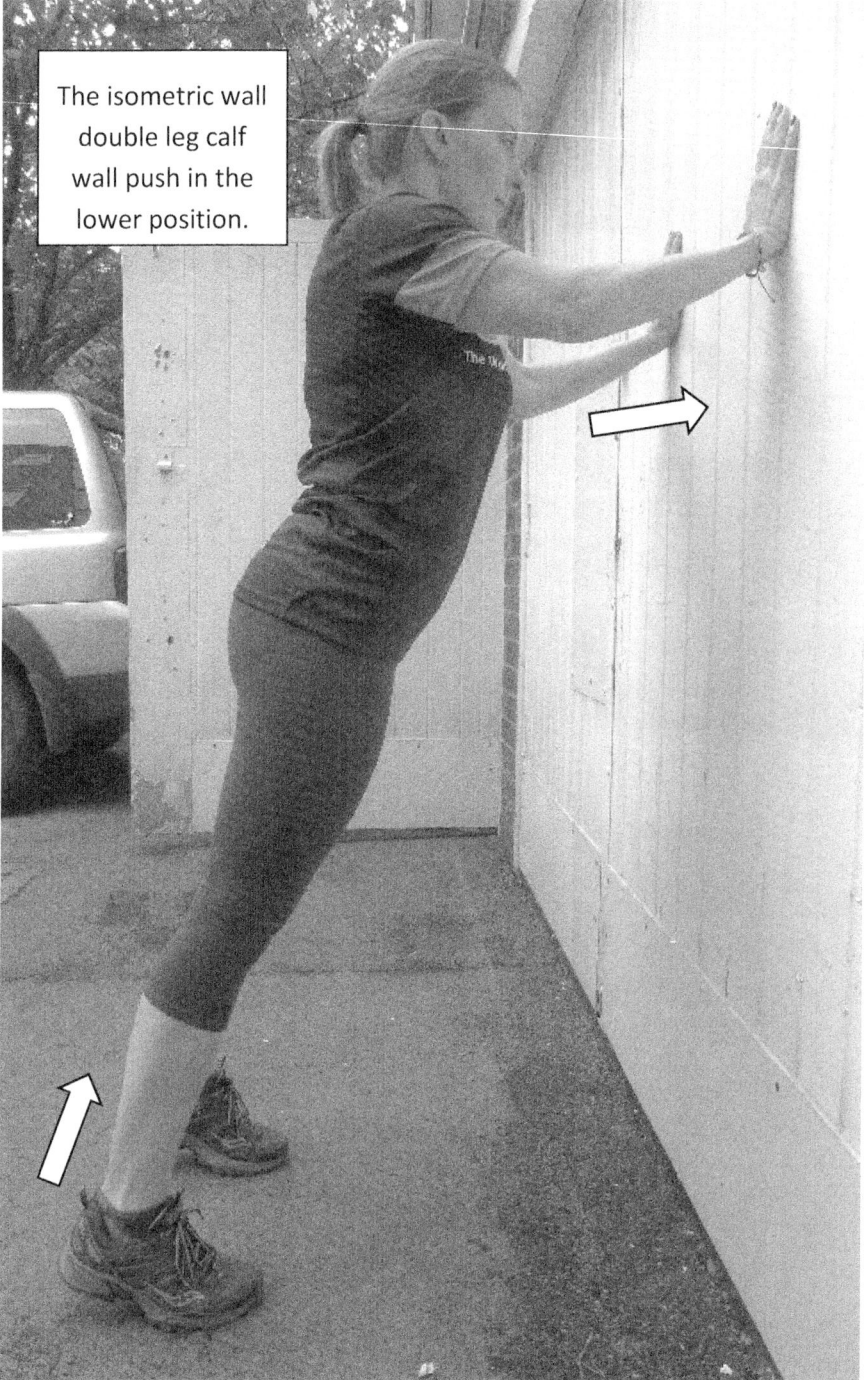

The isometric wall double leg calf wall push in the lower position.

The three positions of the isometric calf wall push.

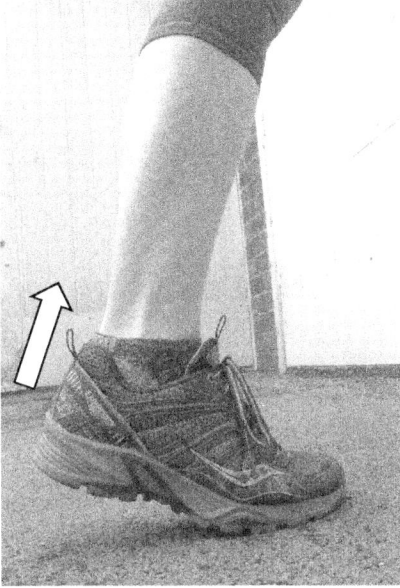

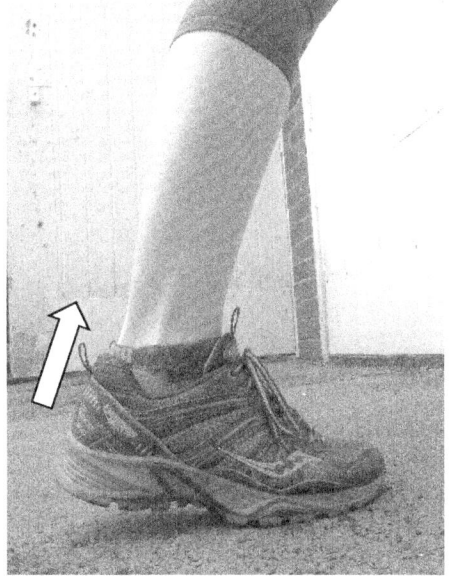

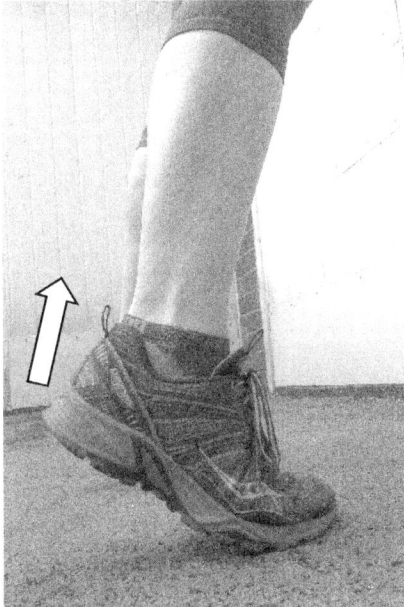

B) Isotonic Double Heel Raise

In the same position, keep your fingertips on the wall or door to aid your balance.

In this position, slowly raise both heels from the floor to the highest point you can reach, pause for a second and then return to the starting position, pause, and repeat.

The exercise should be performed in super-slow style with each portion of the exercise (eccentric and concentric) taking between 10 and 12 seconds to complete. This makes it extremely challenging by any standards.

Since there is only a limited range of motion that can be performed, it will feel almost like you are performing a sequence of many multi-point short duration isometric exercises as you raise and lower the heels. This is precisely what it should feel like to gain maximum benefit.

Never hold your breath, and a suggested method of breathing during super-slow repetitions is to breathe in and out one full breath for each second of elapsed time.

Aim to perform one set of three repetitions, but do not be surprised if you can only manage one at super-slow speed. If this is your limit, even only one repetition performed at super-slow speed will deliver all the results you desire.

Do not sacrifice good exercise style and true super-slow speed in exchange for a greater number of repetitions at a faster speed.

You will gradually increase the number of repetitions you can perform by following the science and adhering to a strict exercise style and good technique.

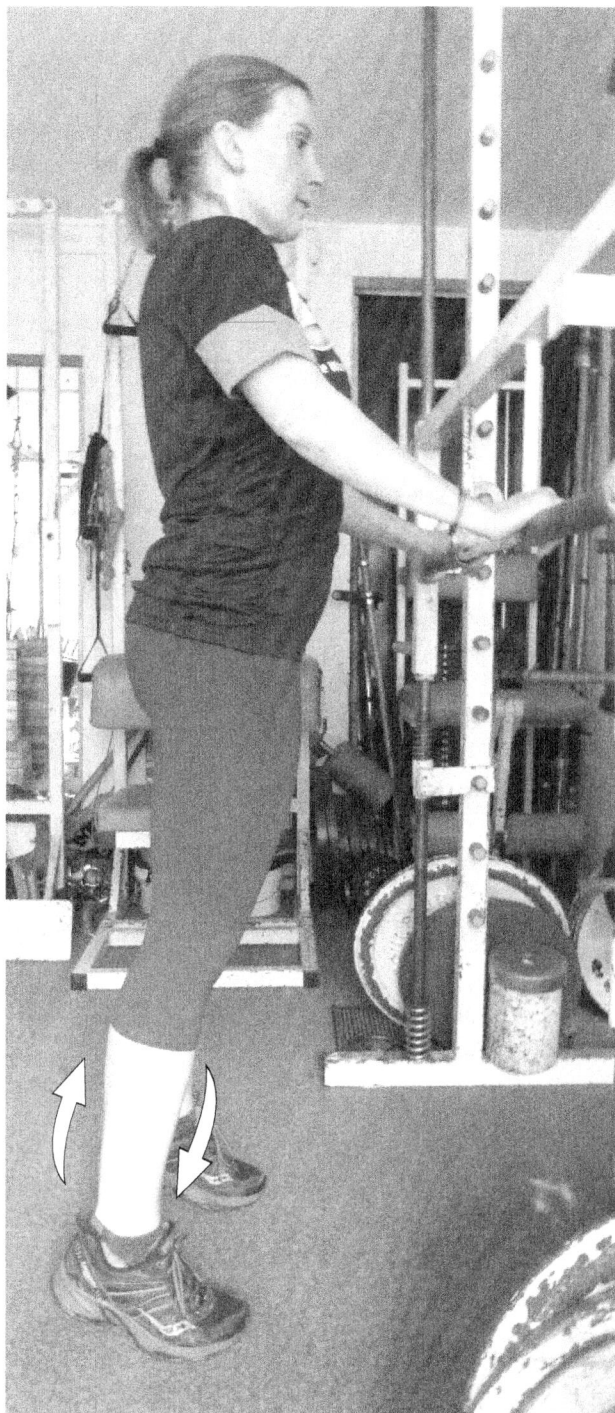

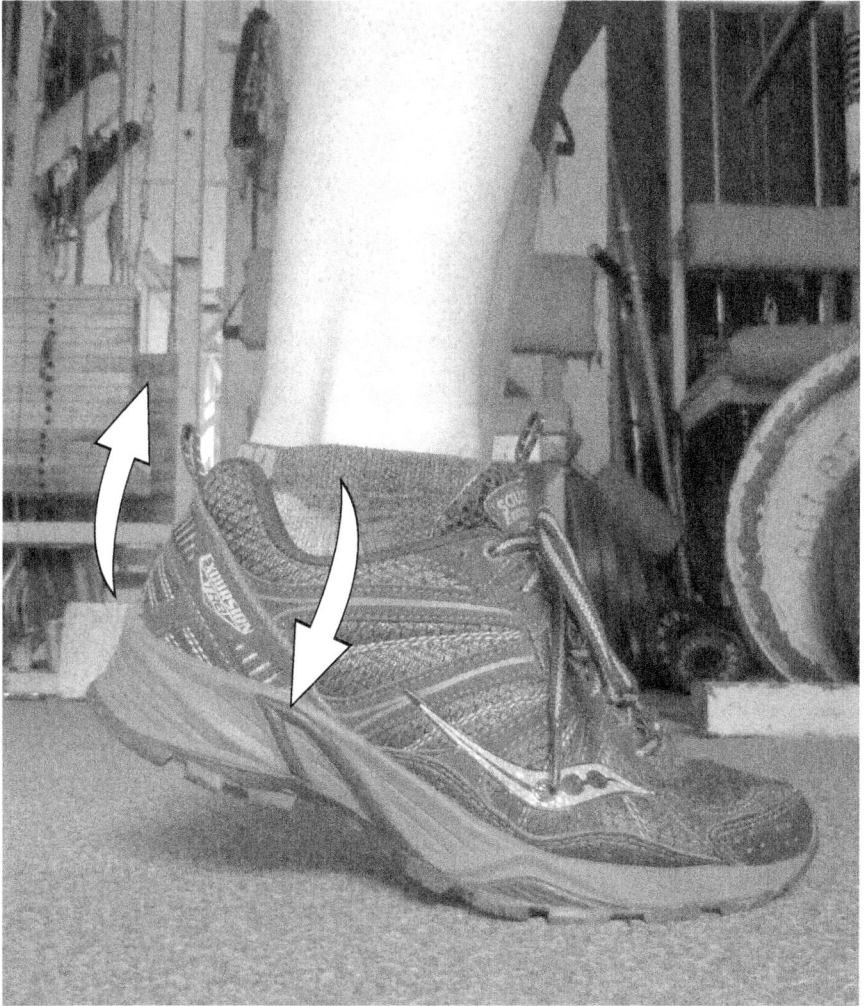

2. Triceps

A) Isometric Triceps Push Down (Rope / Iso-Gym® / Towel / Doorway Pull-Up Bar / Door) *(Triple Position)*

First, decide each of the angles you will assume when performing the three successive isometric exercises. Decide if you will use any equipment or not, and if so, what it will be.

We suggest that you use either the end of a solid bench or a doorway pull-up bar together with a rope of suitable length. Stand in front of a doorway pull-up bar that has been set at an appropriate height to perform the exercises.

Wrap the rope over the doorway pull-up bar and hold the rope by looping it securely around each hand. Keep the arms close to the body with them bent at the elbow and assume the first isometric exercise position.

Gradually apply pressure using Dynamic Flexation™ until you have reached the target level of intensity, then begin the first isometric exercise.

When you perform an isometric exercise never hold your breath. Always breathe deeply and naturally, which will be about 10 full breaths in and out at a rate of about 1 second per full breath. Perform each exercise for no less than 7 seconds, and no longer than 10.

Try not to rest between each exercise for longer than 10 seconds, which should allow enough time to recover while getting into the next position.

Once you have assumed the next isometric exercise angle, perform the exercise in the same way as the previous one, and then perform the third angle isometric exercise in the same way.

With the triple isometric portion of the exercise completed, try to rest for no longer than 10 seconds before performing the isotonic phase.

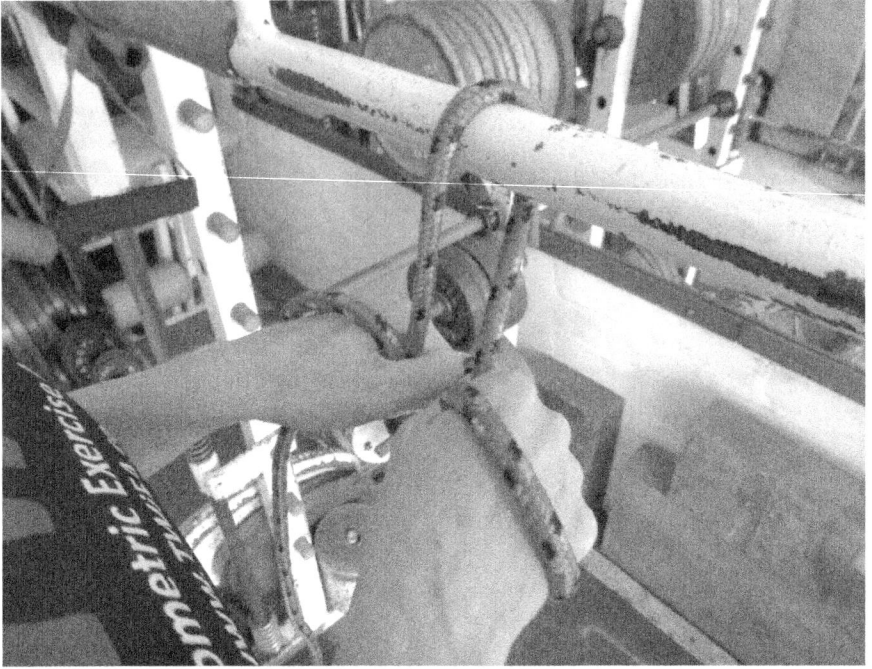

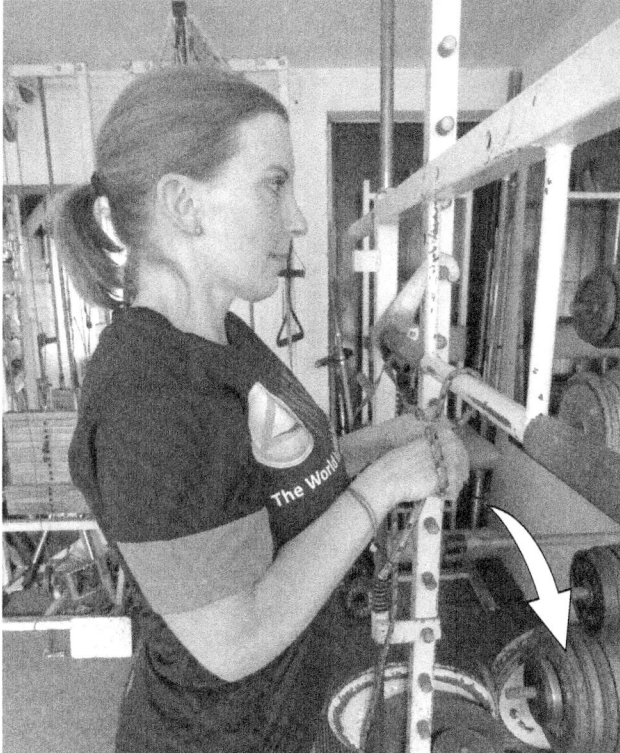

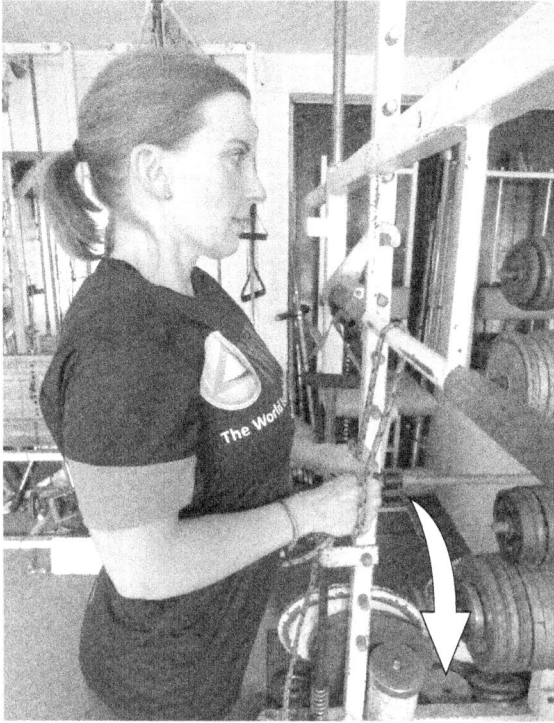

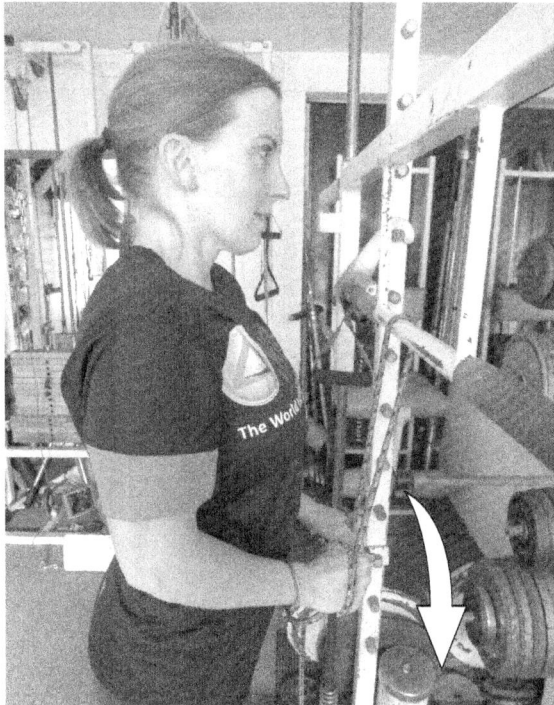

B) Isotonic Triceps 20 to 40 Degree Front Press (Table / Wall / Doorway Pull-up Bar etc.)

Place your hands about 6 inches (15.24 cm) apart on either a wall, a heavy piece of furniture or a doorway pull-up bar. Assume an approximate body angle of between 20 and 40 degrees, which is lower than during the previous routines.

The lower the body angle makes with the bar, the greater the resistance. The higher the bar is positioned, the easier the exercise becomes. The more acute the angle your elbow is placed in, the harder the exercise will be. If you are using a doorway pull-up bar, make certain that it is properly secured to support your bodyweight. If in any doubt do not use it, choose another prop instead.

Starting with your arms fully extended, bend your elbows keeping them close to the body until you have lowered yourself to a point just before your upper chest touches the bar or wall etc. Pause for a second, then return to the starting position to repeat the exercise.

The exercise should be performed in super-slow style with each portion of the exercise (eccentric and concentric) taking between 10 and 12 seconds to complete. This makes it extremely challenging by any standards.

Never hold your breath, and a suggested method of breathing during super-slow repetitions is to breathe in and out one full breath for each second of elapsed time.

Aim to perform one set of three repetitions, but do not be surprised if you can only manage one repetition at super-slow speed. If this is your limit, even only one repetition performed at super-slow speed will deliver all the results you desire.

Do not sacrifice good exercise style and true super-slow speed in exchange for a greater number of repetitions at a faster speed. You will gradually increase the number of repetitions you can perform by following the science and adhering to a strict exercise style and technique.

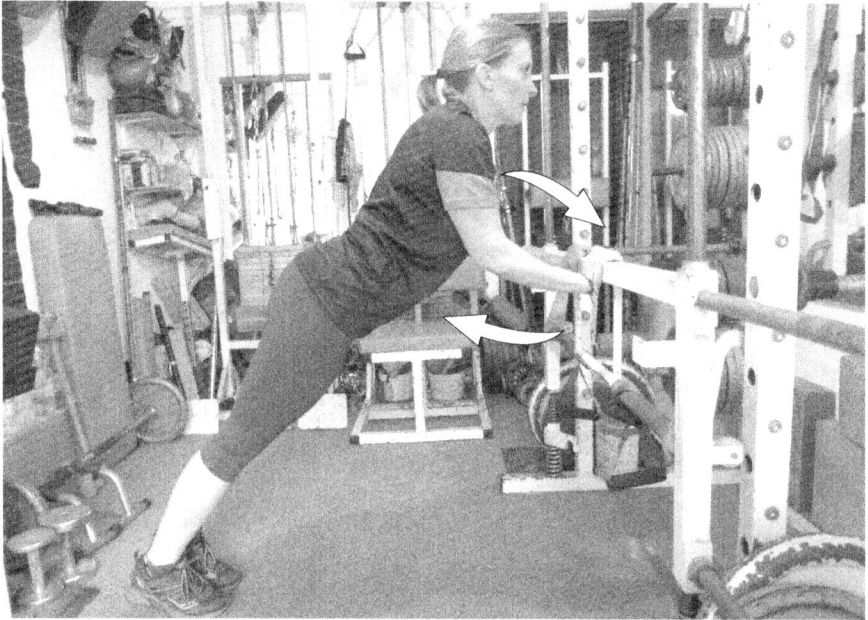

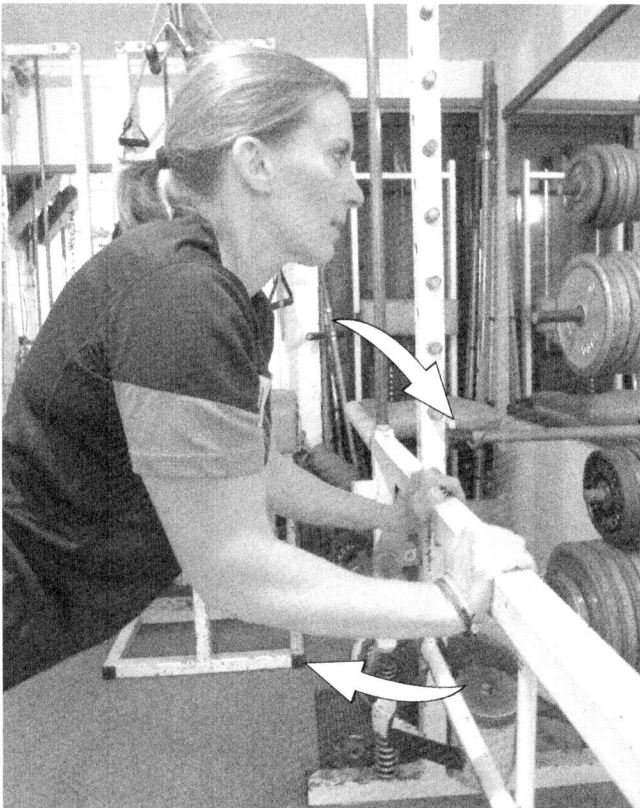

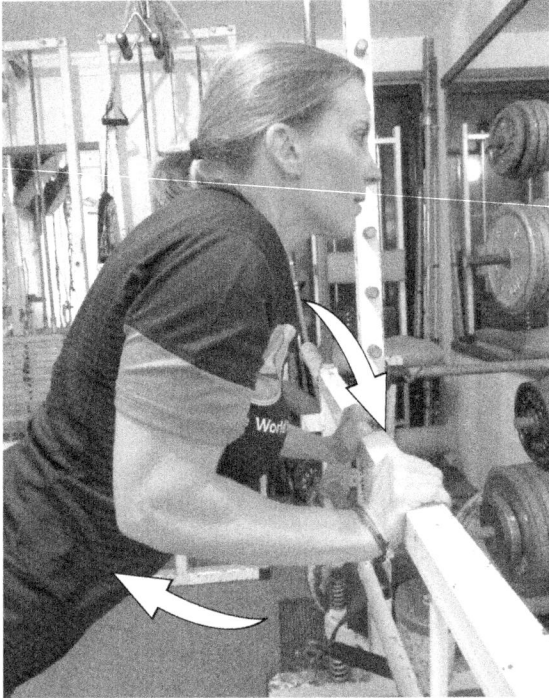
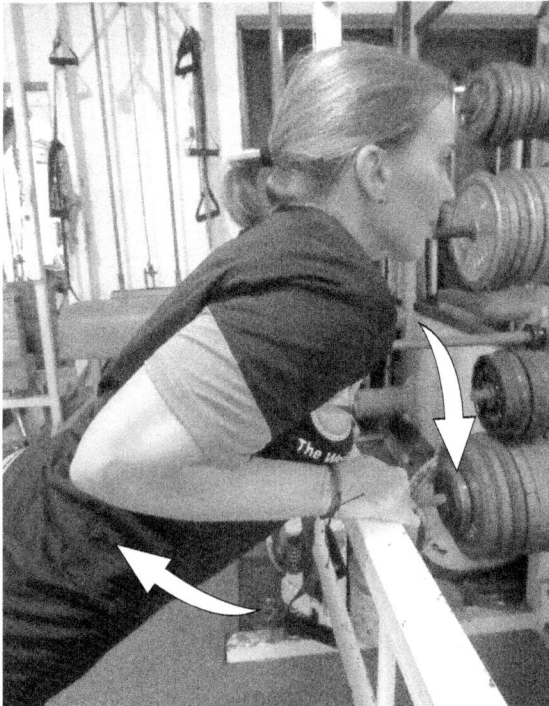

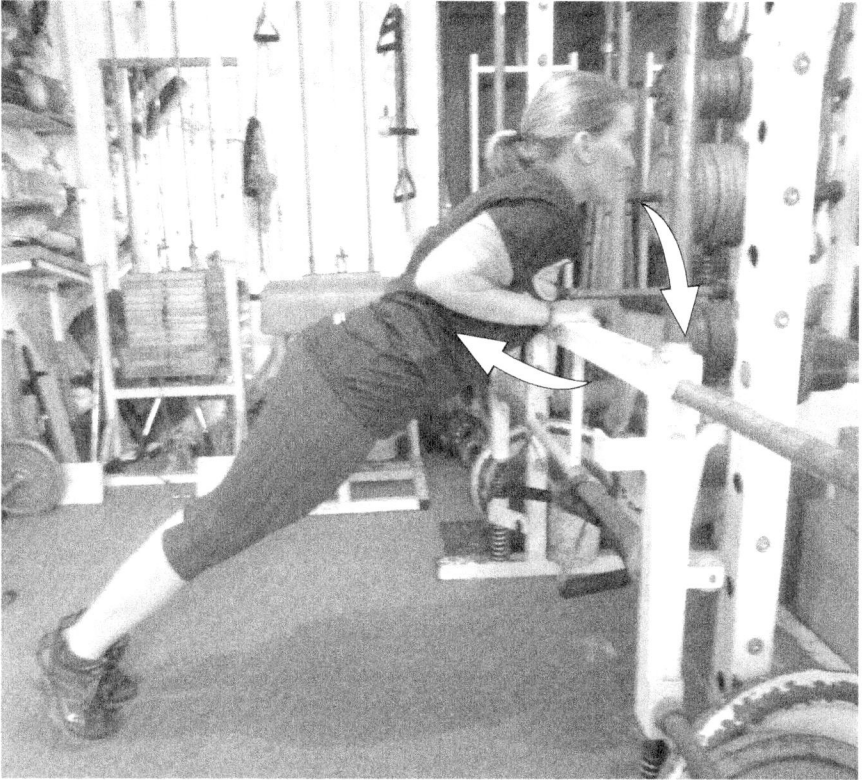

3. Biceps

A) Isometric Doorway Pull-up Bar Biceps Curl (Mid to High Angle Position) (Triple Position Hold) (Grip Either Bar or 2 Looped Iso-Bows®)

First, decide each of the angles you will assume when performing the three successive isometric exercises. Decide what equipment you will use as a bar. We suggest using two Iso-Bows® because this allows a degree of supination to take place as well as making the exercise much more comfortable to perform.

Position a doorway pull-up bar at an appropriate height to provide the right bodyweight resistance for you. The highest position the bar should be is approximately shoulder height. The higher the bar, the easier the exercise will be to perform. The lower the bar, until you are in an almost horizontal suspended position a fraction off the floor at full arm stretch, then the harder the exercises will be.

We suggest starting in a position so that when you are suspended hanging under the bar your body will be at an angle of about 45 degrees. Naturally, you should make any adjustments necessary to make the exercise as easy or as challenging as you need it to be. Loop and interlock a handle through the other side of both Iso-Bow® handles as you wrap them around the doorway pull-up bar. Position each Iso-Bow® at about shoulder-width apart on the bar. Grip each Iso-Bow® handle firmly as you suspend yourself under the doorway pull-up bar. Keep your body straight with your legs and feet forwards so you rest on your heels where they touch the floor.

Move into the first isometric exercise position by performing a curling motion as you apply pressure using Dynamic Flexation™ until you have reached the target level of intensity, then begin the first isometric exercise. When you perform an isometric exercise never hold your breath. Always breathe deeply and naturally, which will be about 10 full breaths in and out at a rate of about 1 second per full breath. Perform each exercise for no less than 7 seconds, and no longer than 10.

Try not to rest between each exercise for longer than 10 seconds, which should allow enough time to recover while getting into the next position. Once you have assumed the next isometric exercise angle, perform the exercise in the same way as the previous one, and then perform the third angle isometric exercise in the same way. With the triple isometric portion of the overall exercise complete, try to rest for no longer than 10 seconds as you move into performing the isotonic phase.

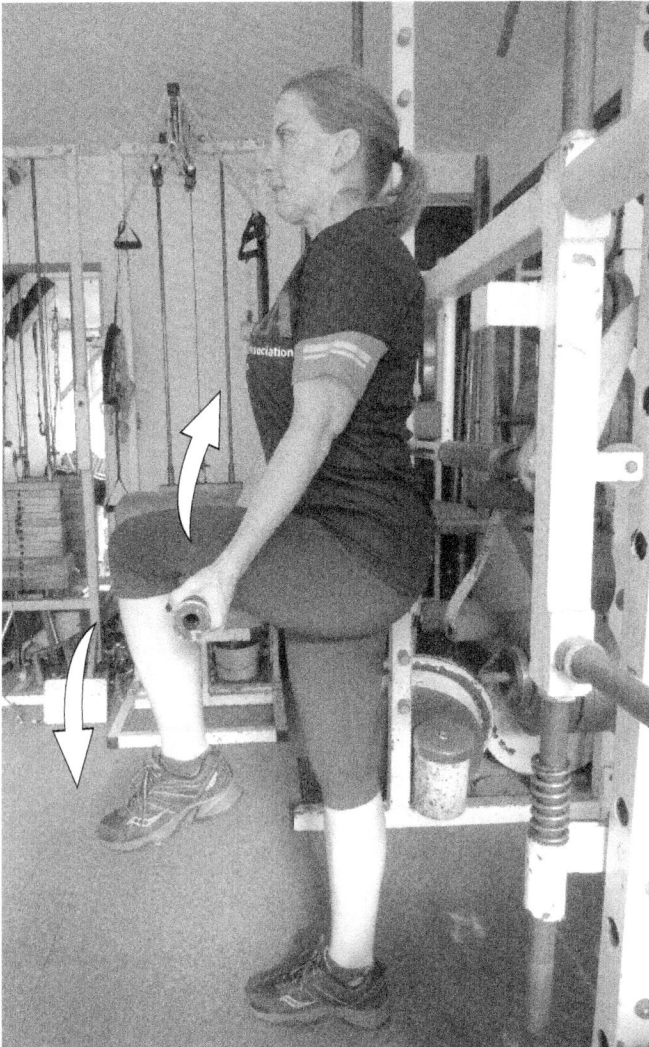

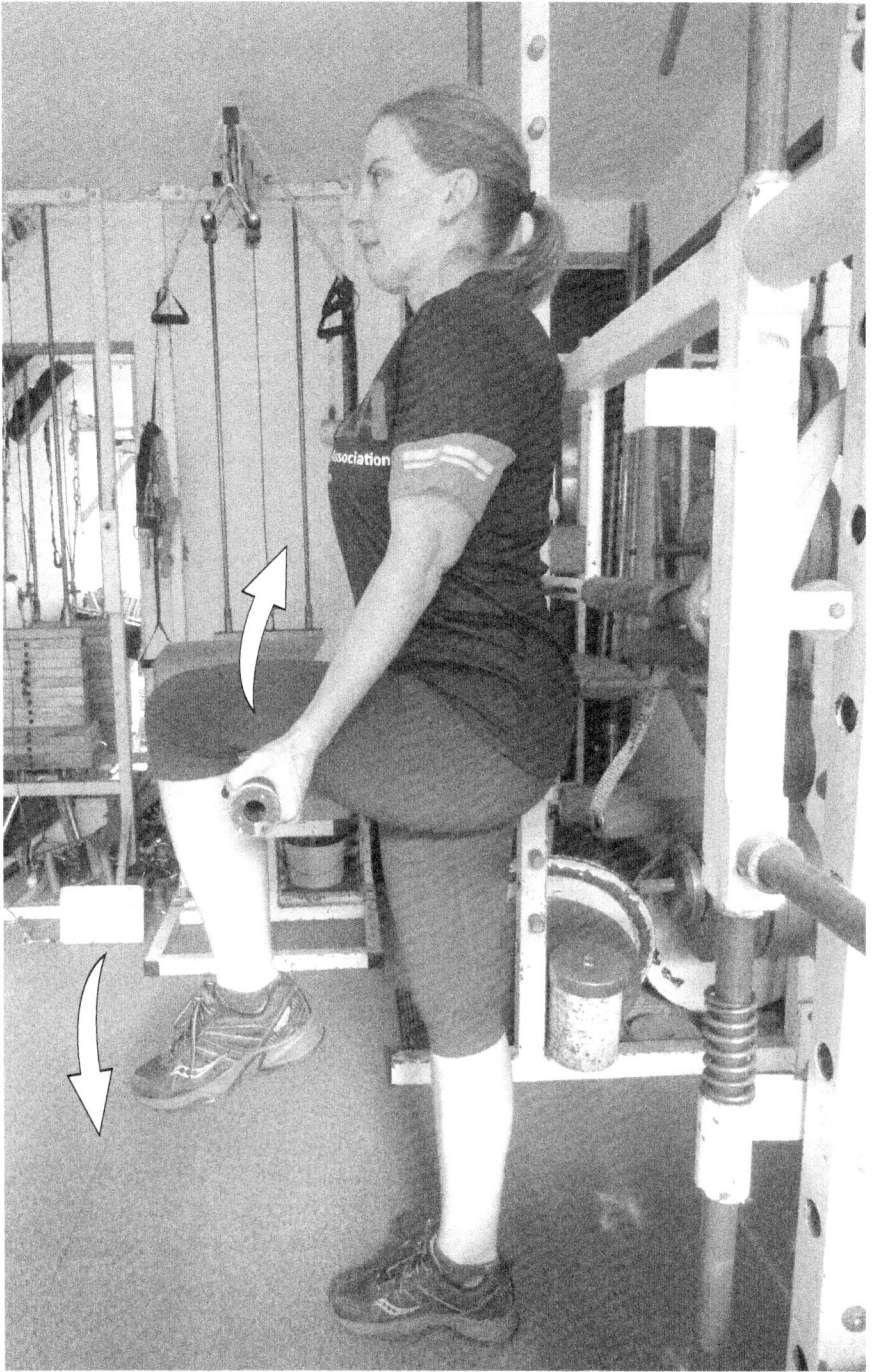

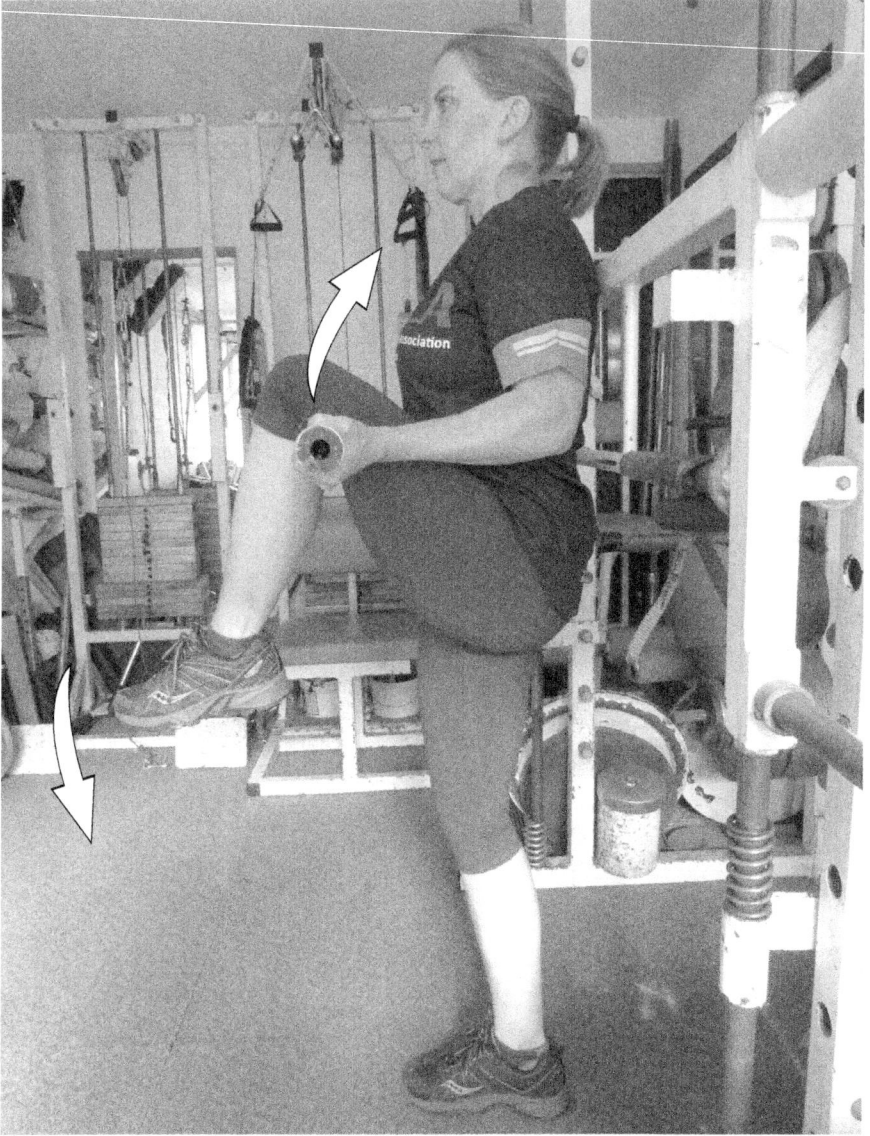

B) Isotonic Doorway Pull-up Bar Biceps Curl (Mid to High Angle Position) (Grip Either Bar or 2 Looped Iso-Bows®)

Continuing with the same exercise position from the completed isometric phase.

Perform the biceps curl in the same way until you reach the top part of the movement, pause, and then return to the starting position to repeat the exercise.

The exercise should be performed in super-slow style with each portion of the exercise (eccentric and concentric) taking between 10 and 12 seconds to complete. This makes it extremely challenging by any standards.

Never hold your breath, and a suggested method of breathing during super-slow repetitions is to breathe in and out one full breath for each second of elapsed time.

Aim to perform one set of three repetitions, but do not be surprised if you can only manage one repetition at super-slow speed. If this is your limit and only one repetition is performed at super-slow speed then it will deliver all the results you desire.

Do not sacrifice good exercise style and true super-slow speed in exchange for a greater number of repetitions at a faster speed.

You will gradually increase the number of repetitions you can perform by following the science and adhering to a strict exercise style and good technique.

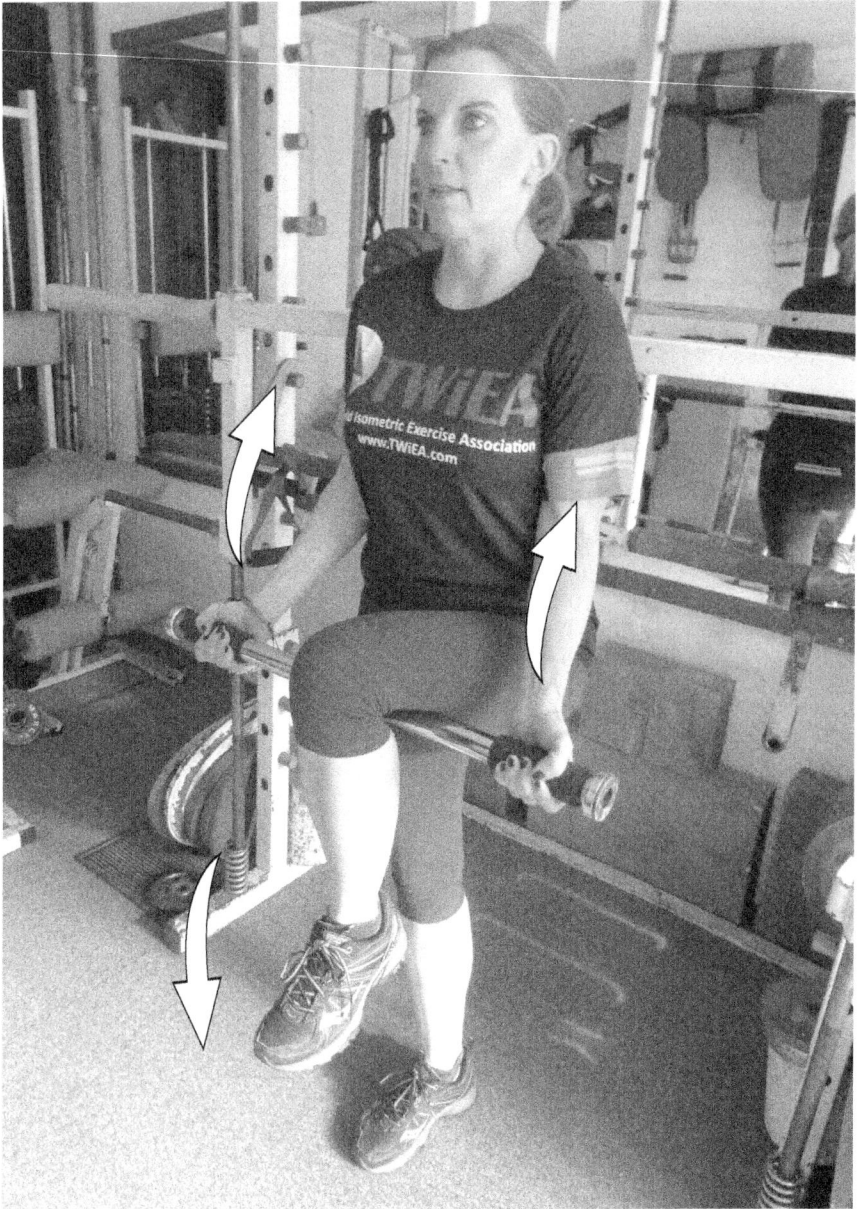

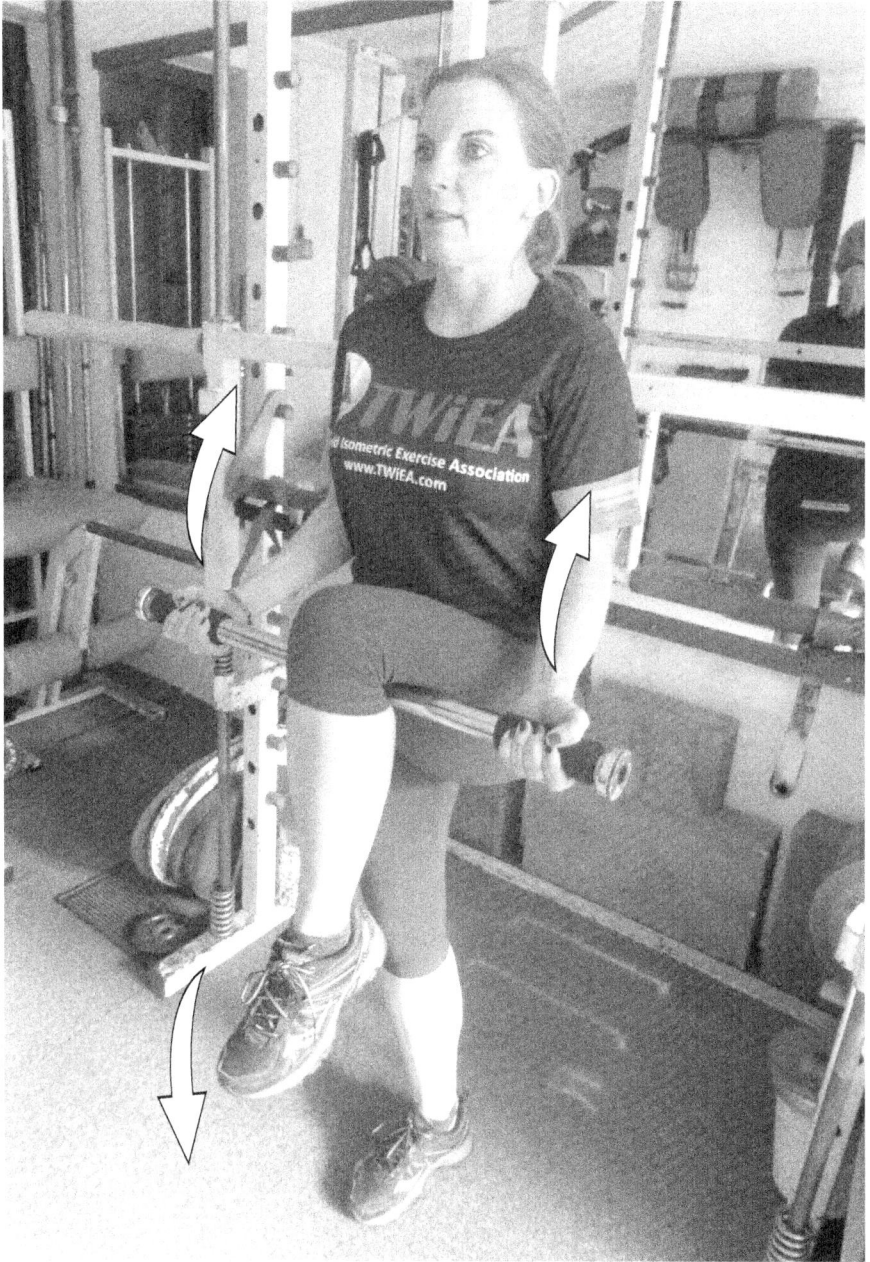

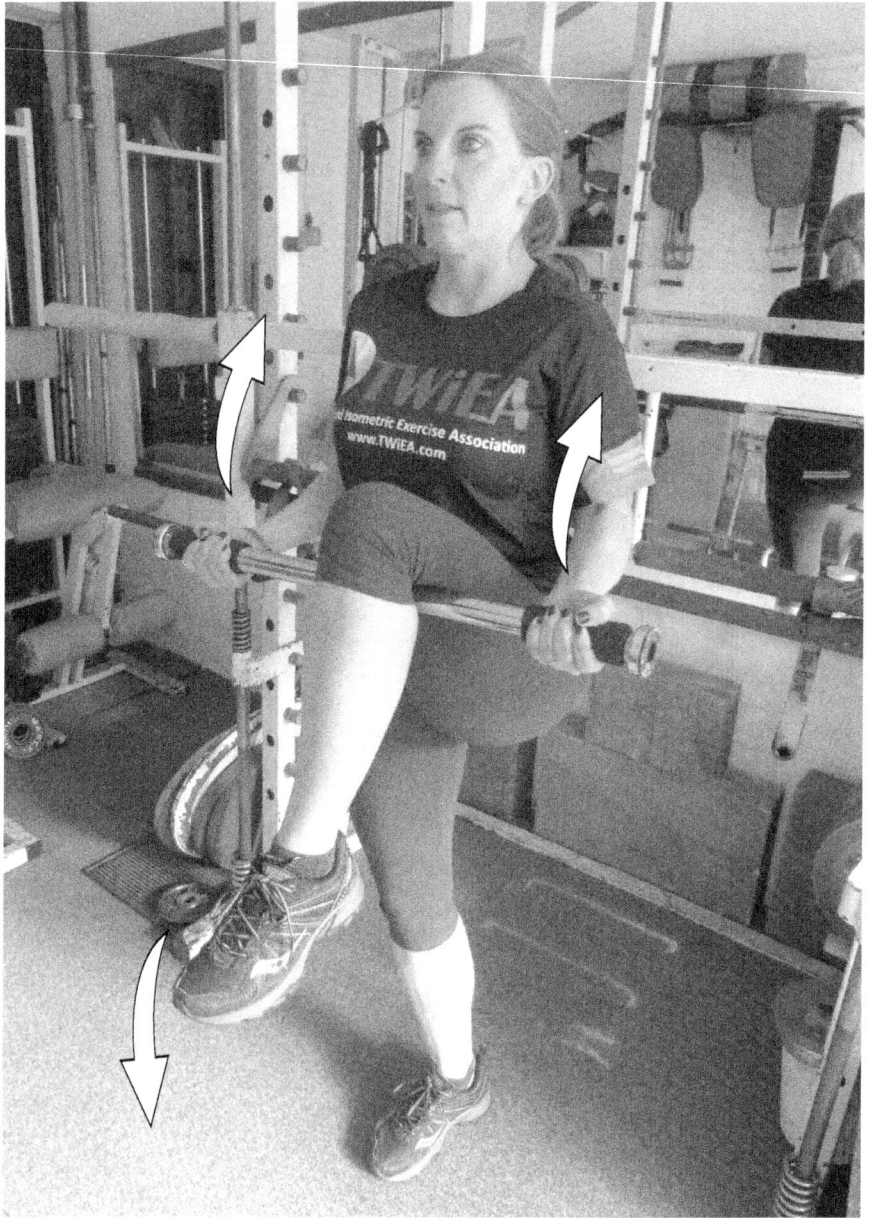

6) Abdominal Set 1 <u>Isometric</u> Bent-Knee Crunch (Triple Position Hold) (Hands/Arms Resisted)

First, decide each of the angles to perform the three successive isometric exercises. Then decide if you will use any equipment or not, and if so, what. If you are, then deploy and test it in advance of beginning both exercise phases, even if it will only be used for just one of the phases. Lie back on the floor with both knees bent and your feet flat on the floor about shoulder-width apart. Place your arms with clenched fists together in front of your chest and stomach, so your fists sit just under your chin to support your neck and head. Contract your abdominals and curl your body upwards as if you are slowly peeling it from the floor fractionally with your shoulders leading. It should feel as though you are beginning to curl yourself and wrap around a large ball. Keep your lower back flat on the floor, and the highest point of the exercise is always just before the lower back is about to rise. There is a limited range of motion in this exercise and never allow yourself to begin performing a full sit up. Once you are in the first isometric exercise position, hold at that point. In this position, gradually apply pressure using Dynamic Flexation™ until you have applied the approximate desired target level of force, then begin. When you perform an isometric exercise never hold your breath. Always breathe deeply and naturally, which will be about 10 full breaths in and out at a rate of about 1 second per full breath. Perform each exercise for no less than 7 seconds, and no longer than 10. Try not to rest between each exercise for longer than 10 seconds, which should allow enough time to recover while getting into the next position. Once you have assumed the next isometric exercise angle, perform the exercise in the same way as previously and perform the third angle isometric exercise in the same way. With the triple isometric portion of the exercise completed, try to rest for no longer than 10 seconds before performing the isotonic phase. **NOTE:** If necessary, secure your feet or knees to prevent your lower body from rising as you curl your torso during the exercise. This will help you to focus more on better exercise style and targeting the right muscles.

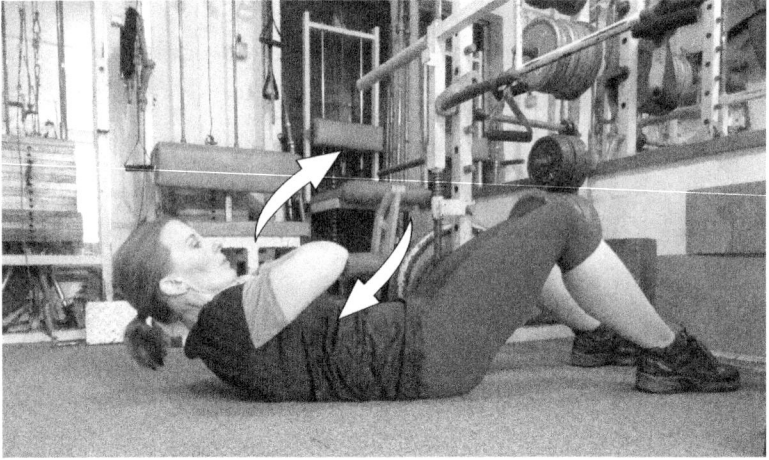
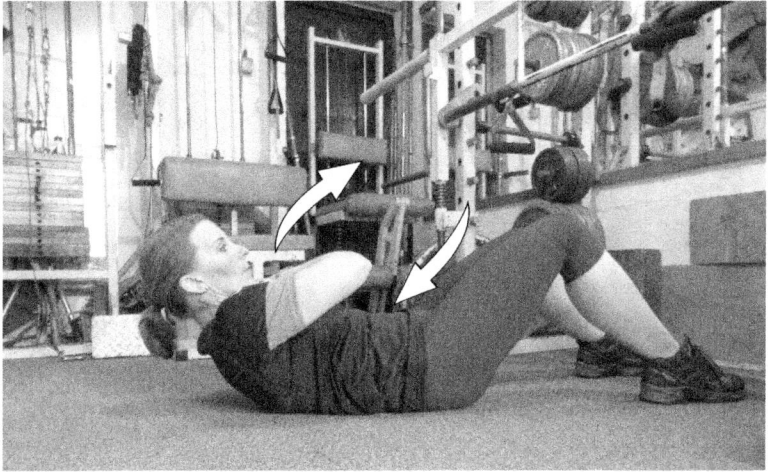
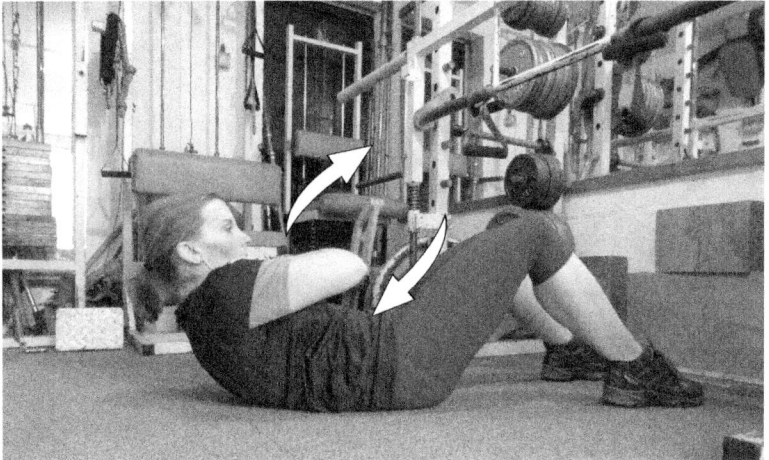

6. Abdominal Set 1 <u>Isotonic</u> Bent-Knee Crunch (Hands/Arms Resisted)

Maintain the same position as the isometric phase of the exercise, with your back and feet flat on the floor and your knees bent. Perform the body curling action in the same way, however, do not stop and hold until you reach the natural top of the movement. At that point, you pause and then slowly return to the starting position to repeat the exercise.

As you curl up you can provide additional resistance by pushing against the torso-curling action using your hands and arms pushing against your upper thighs.

The exercise should be performed in super-slow style with each portion of the exercise (eccentric and concentric) taking between 10 and 12 seconds to complete. This makes it extremely challenging by any standards.

Never hold your breath, and a suggested method of breathing during super-slow repetitions is to breathe in and out one full breath for each second of elapsed time.

Aim to perform one set of three repetitions, but do not be surprised if you can only manage one repetition at super-slow speed. If this is your limit, even only one or two repetitions performed at super-slow speed will deliver all the results you desire.

Do not sacrifice good exercise style and true super-slow speed in exchange for a greater number of repetitions at a faster speed. You will gradually increase the number of repetitions you can perform by following the science and adhering to a strict exercise style and good technique.

NOTE: If necessary, secure your feet or knees to prevent your lower body from rising off the floor as you curl your torso. This will help you to focus more on better exercise style and targeting the right muscles.

7. Abdominal Set 2 <u>Isometric</u> Kneeling Side Bend (Iso-Bow® Loop Secured Under Each Knee / Rope or Towel under both knees) (Triple Position Hold)

First, decide each of the angles you will assume when performing the three successive isometric exercises. Then decide what equipment you will use and deploy it.

We will assume that you are using a rope for this description. Kneel on the floor or an exercise mat. Place a strong rope of enough length under both knees.

Hold the rope at the correct length and assume your first isometric exercise position on one side of your body.

In this position, gradually apply pressure using Dynamic Flexation™ until you have applied the approximate desired target level of intensity. Then begin the first isometric exercise.

Perform both the isometric and isotonic phases for one side of the body only, once that side has been completed, then you should repeat the sequence on the other side of the body.

When you perform an isometric exercise never hold your breath. Always breathe deeply and naturally, which will be about 10 full breaths in and out at a rate of about 1 second per full breath. Perform each exercise for no less than 7 seconds, and no longer than 10.

Try not to rest between each exercise for longer than 10 seconds, which should allow enough time to recover while getting into the next position.

Once you have assumed the next isometric exercise angle, perform the exercise in the same way as the previous one, and then perform the third angle isometric exercise in the same way.

With the triple isometric portion of the exercise completed, try to rest for no longer than 10 seconds before performing the isotonic phase.

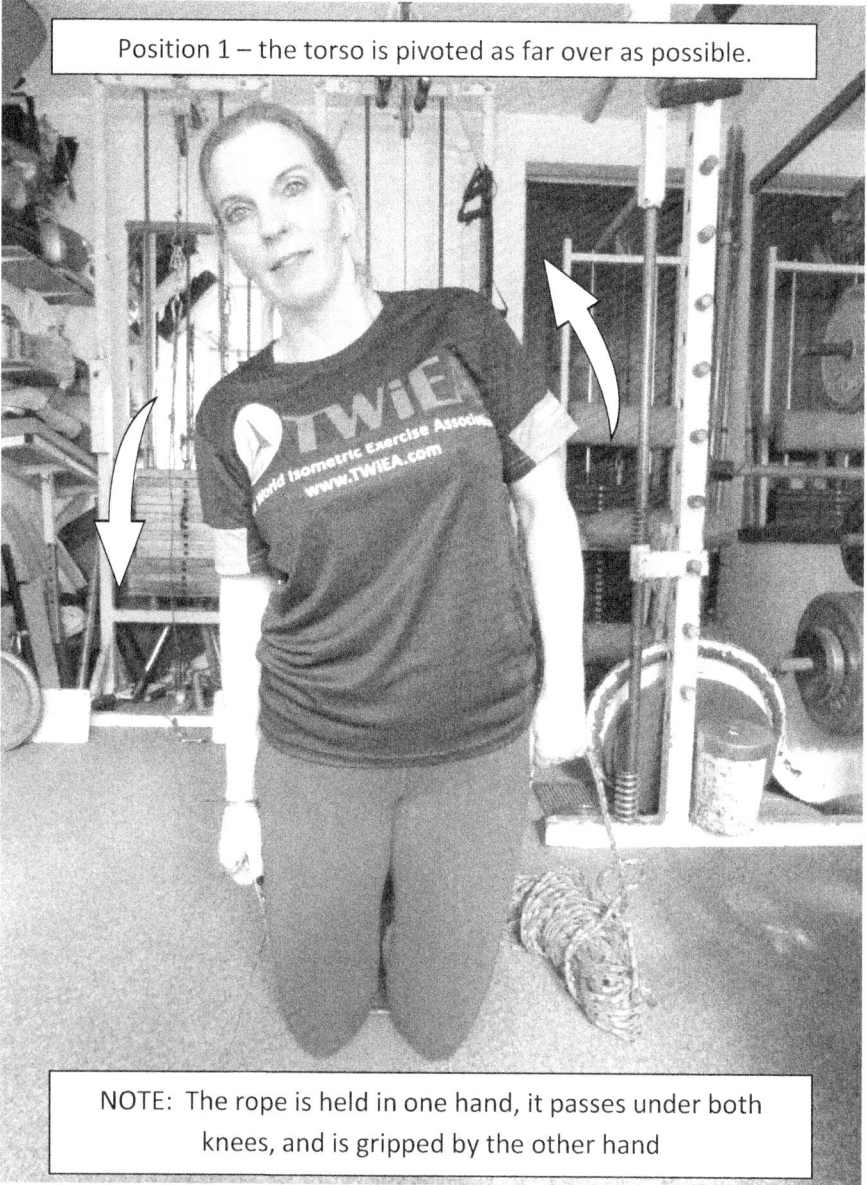

Position 1 – the torso is pivoted as far over as possible.

NOTE: The rope is held in one hand, it passes under both knees, and is gripped by the other hand

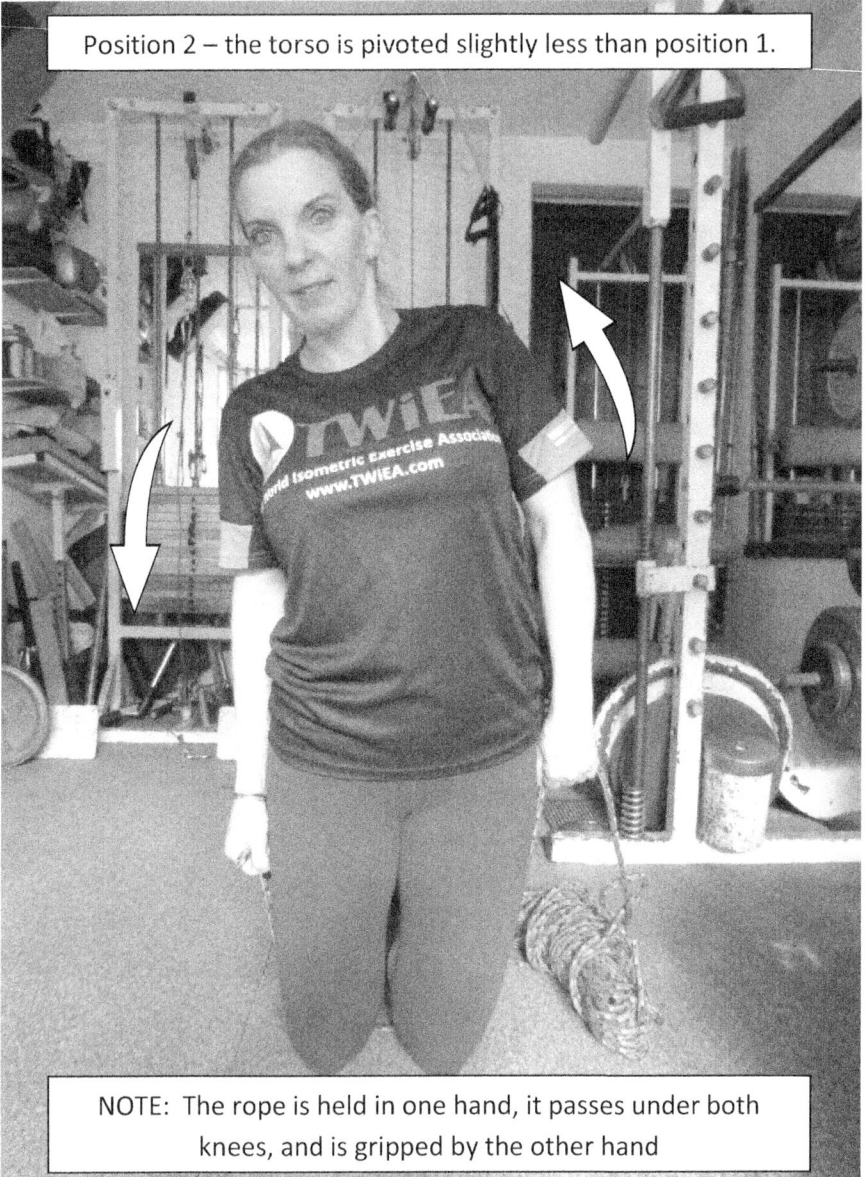

Position 2 – the torso is pivoted slightly less than position 1.

NOTE: The rope is held in one hand, it passes under both knees, and is gripped by the other hand

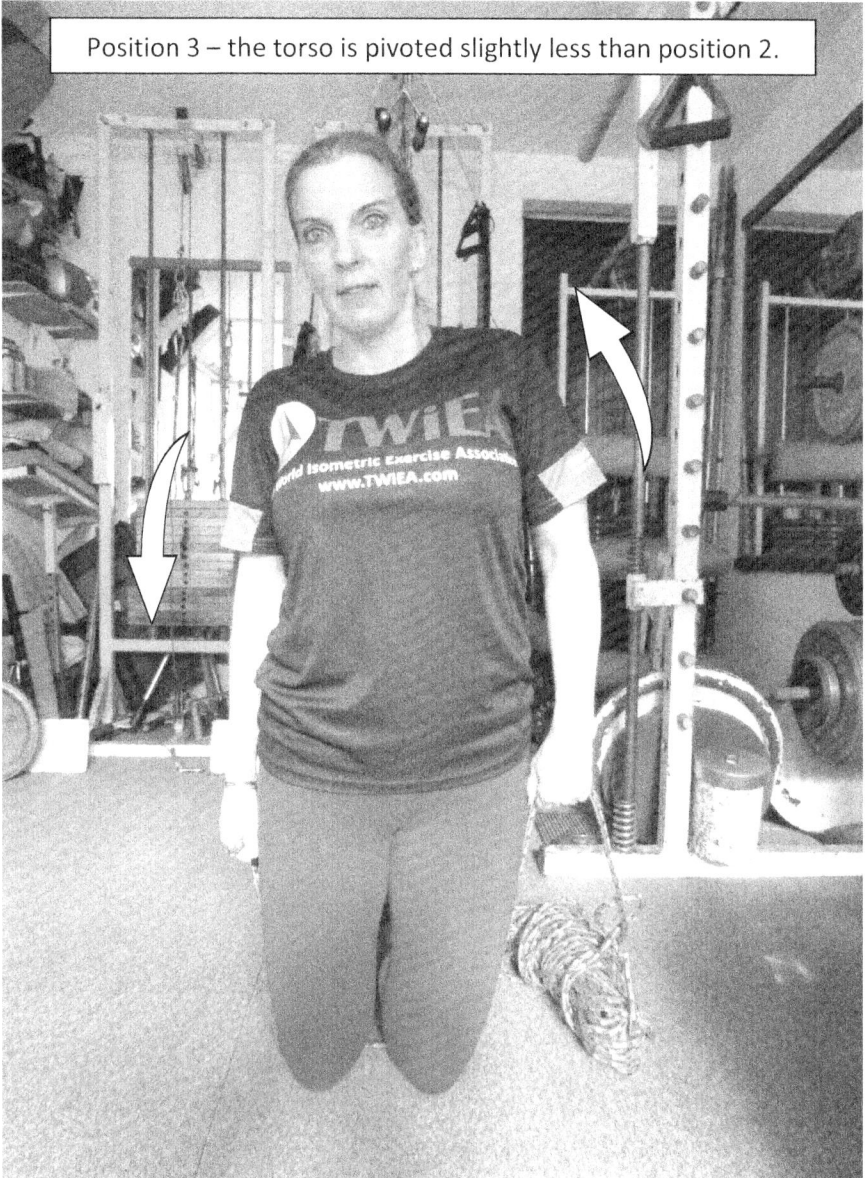

Position 3 – the torso is pivoted slightly less than position 2.

NOTE: The rope is held in one hand, it passes under both knees, and is gripped by the other hand

7. Abdominal Set 2 <u>Isotonic</u> Elbow Supported Side Crunch

Lie sideways on the floor or on an exercise mat. Suspend your body in the side position. this is on one elbow and forearm which will be directly below your shoulder and with the side of your foot. Hold both feet together and form a straight line with the entire body held in the side leaning position. Keep your head and neck straight too.

Maintaining a perfect sideways position, relax your body to allow it to bend sideways from the hips to the lowest comfortable point, pause, and then contract your oblique abdominal and core-supporting muscles to raise your hips back to the starting position with your body in a straight line from head to feet when you can repeat the exercise.

The exercise should be performed in super-slow style with each portion of the exercise (eccentric and concentric) taking between 10 and 12 seconds to complete. This makes it extremely challenging by any standards.

Never hold your breath, and a suggested method of breathing during super-slow repetitions is to breathe in and out one full breath for each second of elapsed time.

Aim to perform one set of three repetitions, but do not be surprised if you can only manage one repetition at super-slow speed. If this is your limit, even only one repetition performed at super-slow speed will deliver all the results you desire.

Do not sacrifice good exercise style and true super-slow speed in exchange for a greater number of repetitions at a faster speed.

You will gradually increase the number of repetitions you can perform by following the science and adhering to a strict exercise style and good technique.

NOTE: Exercise both sides of the body

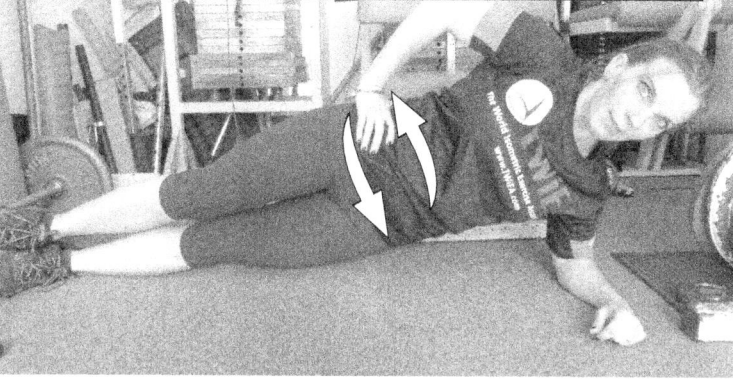
Position 1 The torso is straight.

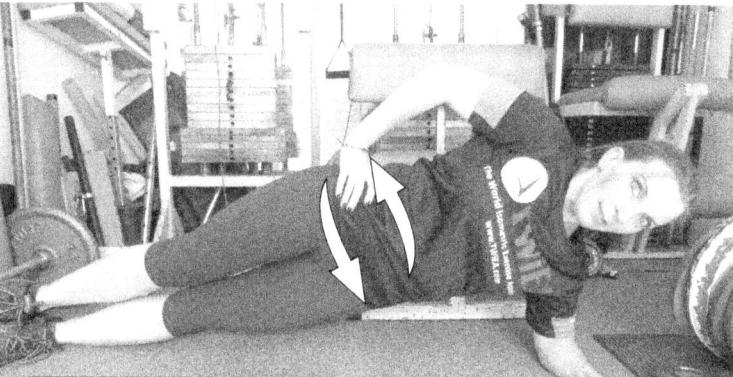
Position 2 The torso is bent sideways slightly more.

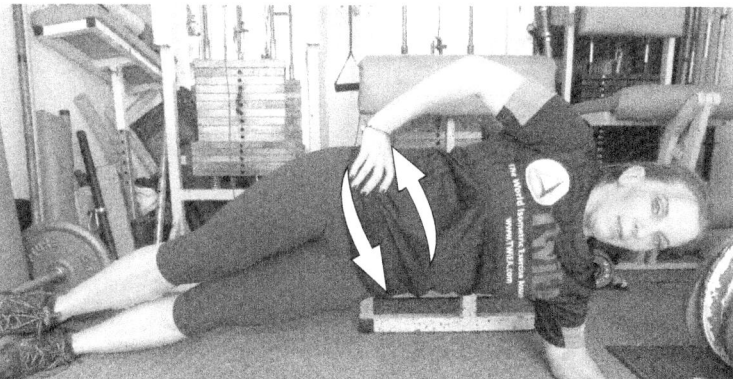
Position 3 The torso is bent sideways even more.

8. Back - Upper

A) Isometric Latissimus Overhead Pull-Apart (Rope / Iso-Bow® / Towel / Hands) (Triple Position Hold)

First, decide each of the angles you will assume when performing the three successive isometric exercises. Then decide if you will use any equipment or not, and if so, what it will be. If you are going to use any equipment then deploy and test it in advance of beginning both the isometric and isotonic exercise phases for this body part, even if it will only be used for just one of the phases.

With your torso upright, raise your bent arms to lock together directly overhead. Use an inter-hook grip with your fingers or any other solid grip that will not slip. If you are using rope or a towel, then make sure you grip it securely. You can loop the rope around your hands if needed. An Iso-Bow® or similar will provide you with the best grip.

Attempt to pull your hands apart in a sideways and downwards direction to the correct position for the first isometric exercise. Your grip prevents your hands from being pulled apart as you engage the upper back muscles as the driving force. Gradually apply pressure using Dynamic Flexation™ until you have applied the approximate desired target level of intensity, then begin the first isometric exercise.

When you perform an isometric exercise never hold your breath. Always breathe deeply and naturally, which will be about 10 full breaths in and out at a rate of about 1 second per full breath. Perform each exercise for no less than 7 seconds, and no longer than 10.

Try not to rest between each exercise for longer than 10 seconds, which should allow enough time to recover while getting into the next position. Once you have assumed the next isometric exercise angle, perform the exercise in the same way as the previous one, and then perform the third angle isometric exercise in the same way.

With the triple isometric portion of the exercise completed, try to rest for no longer than 10 seconds before performing the isotonic phase.

239

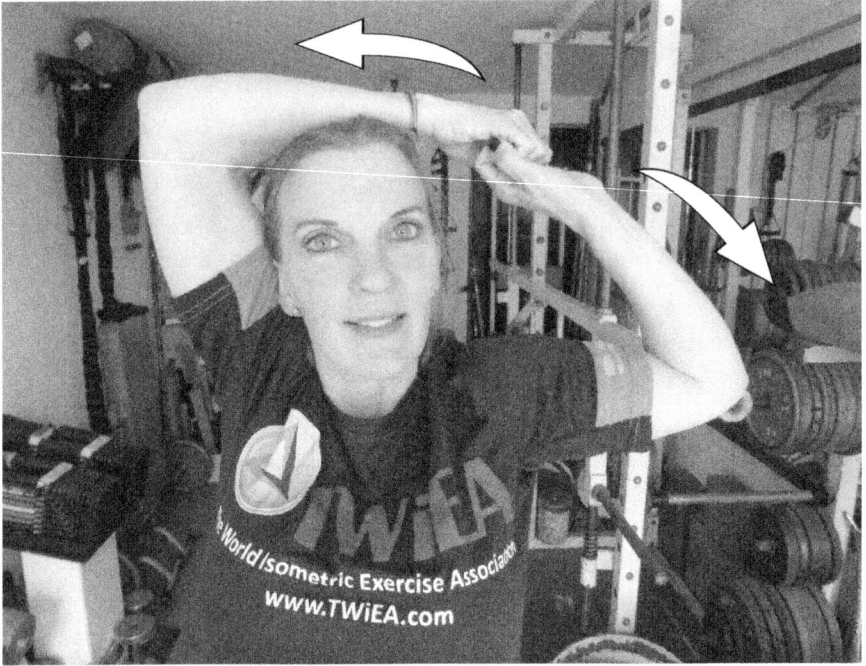
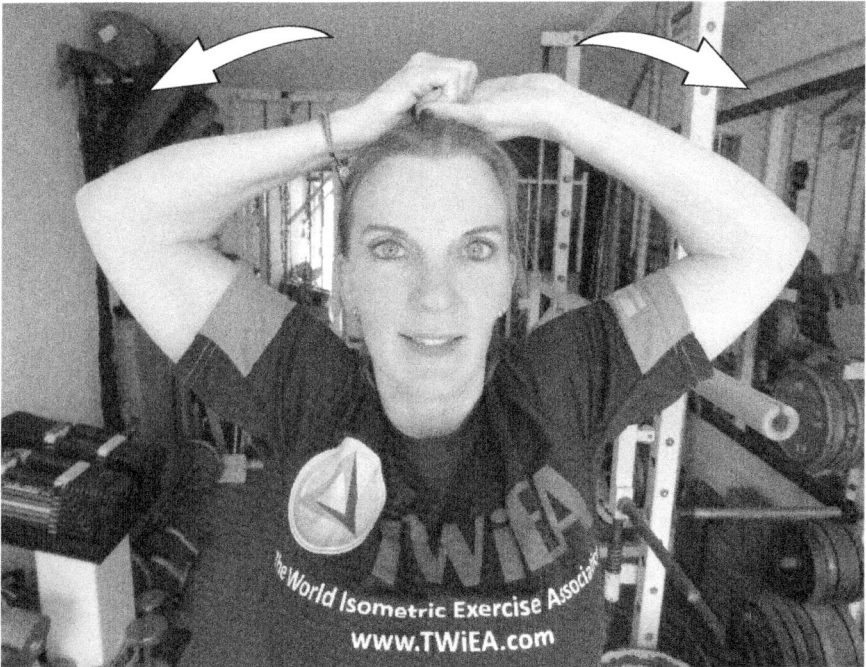

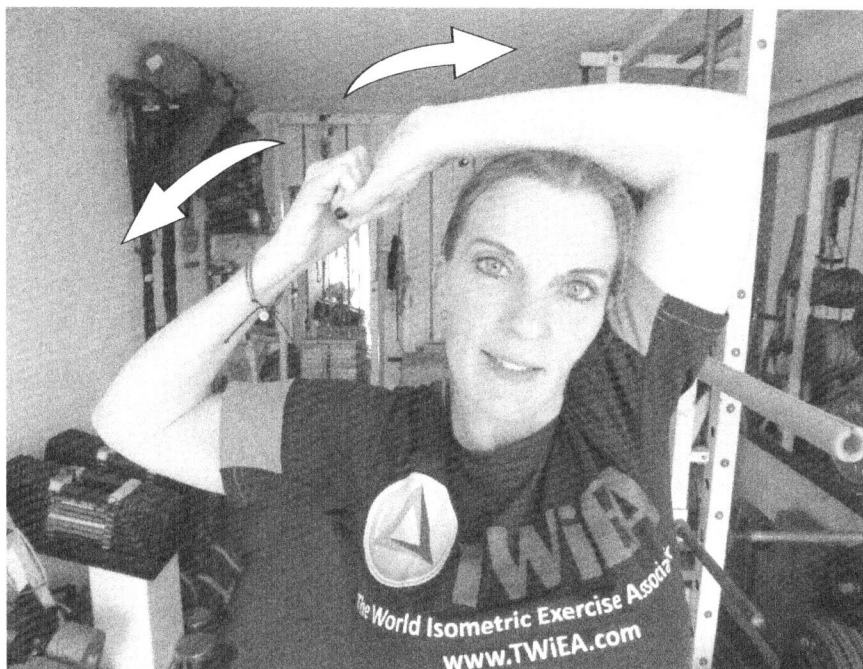

8. Back – Upper
B) Isotonic Seated Pull-ups (Doorway Pull-up Bar)

A doorway pull-up bar, or similar, will be needed to perform this exercise. The bar should be positioned at a height so that when hanging from it at your full arm's length while seated, you are still just very slightly clear of the floor. For the most comfortable handgrip and the best results from the exercise, we highly recommend using 2 Iso-Bows® with each of them looped and interlocked around the bar securely. They should be positioned slightly wider than shoulder-width apart so that at the mid-point of the exercise the forearms and upper arms are at approximately a 90-degree angle. Sit on the floor directly under the bar and suspend yourself from the bar with the heels of your feet on the floor and your body bent into an 'L' shape as you do so. Pull upwards using the upper back muscles as the primary drivers, at the top of the movement pause for a second, and then return to the starting position to repeat the exercise. The exercise should be performed in super-slow style with each portion of the exercise (eccentric and concentric) taking between 10 and 12 seconds to complete. This makes it extremely challenging by any standards. Never hold your breath, and a suggested method of breathing during super-slow repetitions is to breathe in and out one full breath for each second of elapsed time. Aim to perform one set of three repetitions, but do not be surprised if you can only manage one repetition at super-slow speed. If this is your limit, even only one repetition performed at super-slow speed will deliver all the results you desire. Do not sacrifice good exercise style and true super-slow speed in exchange for a greater number of repetitions at a faster speed. You will gradually increase the number of repetitions you can perform by following the science and adhering to a strict exercise style and good technique. **NOTE:** if this exercise is extremely challenging, bend the knees and move the feet closer to your torso and if needed, place your feet flat on the floor. However, offsetting your body weight to reduce the resistance too much will also reduce the results you get from the exercise. Suggested equipment: 2 x Iso-Bows® and 1 x doorway pull-up bar.

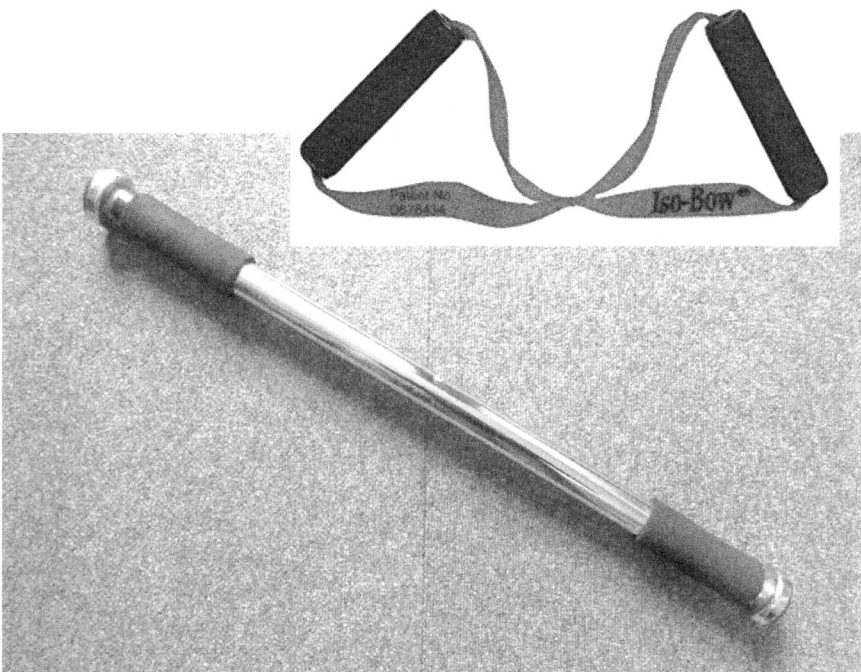

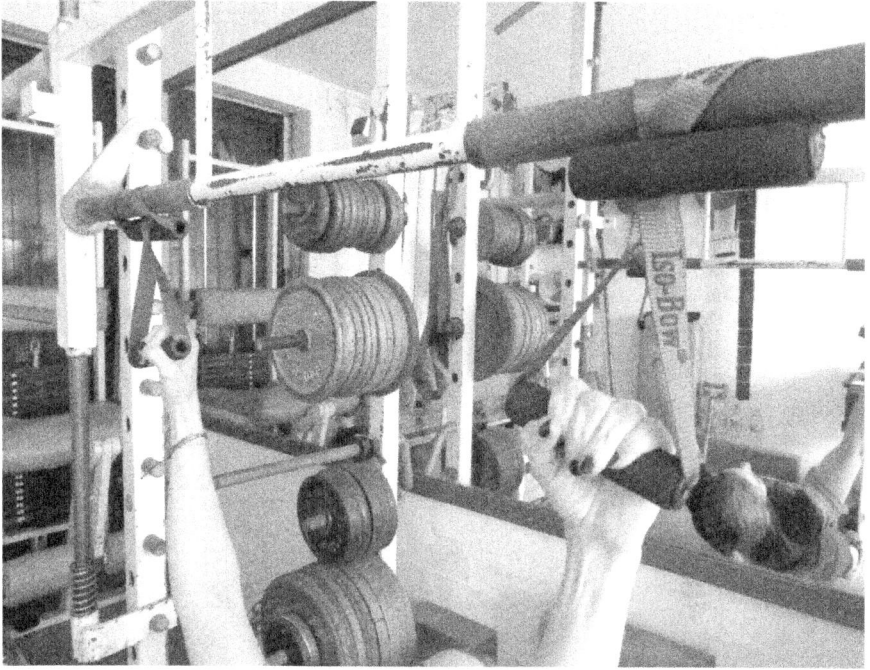

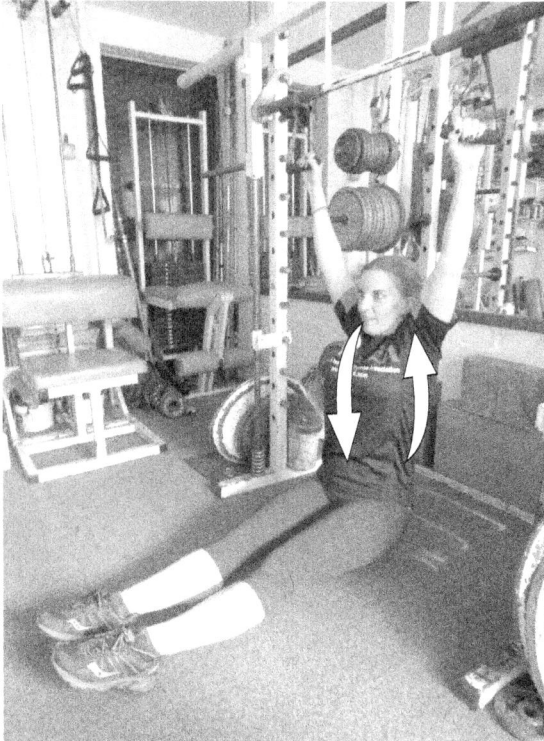

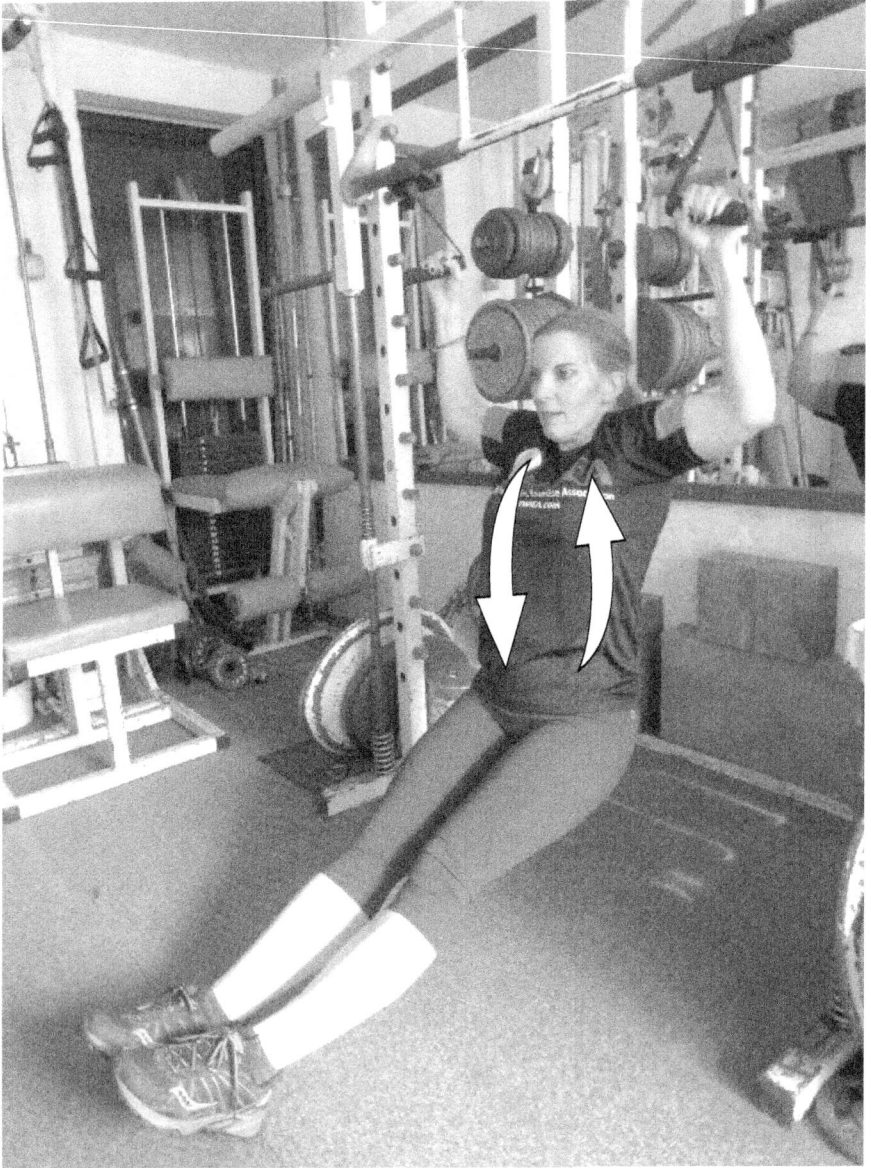

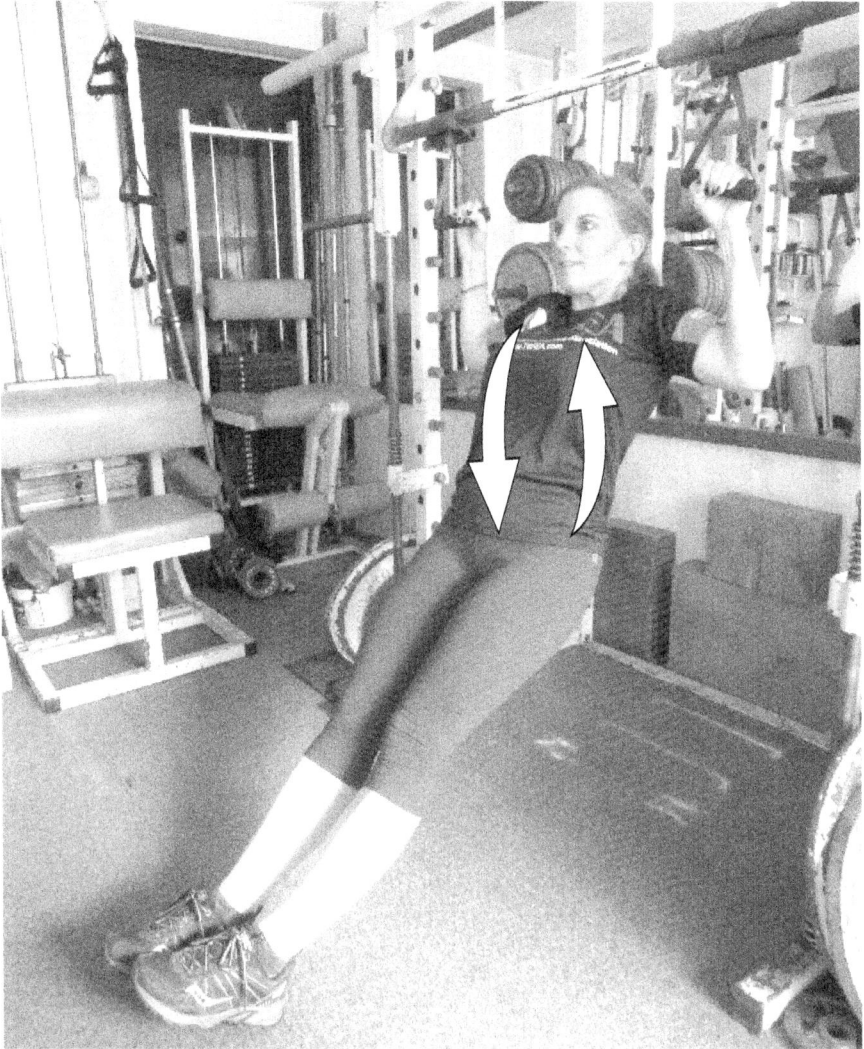

9. **Shoulders (Left Side)**
10. **Shoulders (Right Side)**
A) **Isometric Front Raise (Left and Right Side) (Rope / Iso-Bow® / Towel / Hand) (Triple Position Hold)**

First, decide each of the angles you will assume when performing the three successive isometric exercises. Then decide if you will use any equipment or not, and if so, what it will be.

If you are going to use any equipment then deploy and test it in advance of beginning both the isometric and isotonic exercise phases for this body part, even if it will only be used for just one of the phases.

We will assume that you are using your hands to perform the exercise, instead of equipment.

Stand upright with your arms hanging at full length in front of you. Make a fist with one hand and place the palm of the other hand over it, to wrap around the back of the clenched fist hand.

At this point, very slightly bend the elbows of both arms and keep them in this slightly bent locked position throughout the exercise. This will reduce any unnecessary exercise stress being placed on the elbow joints.

The arm with the clenched fist will be one exercising the front deltoid muscles, the arm with the open hand will serve as the resistance.

Raise the arm with the clenched fist to the first isometric exercise position as you engage the front deltoid of one arm as the driving force.

Gradually apply pressure using Dynamic Flexation™ until you have applied the approximate desired target level of intensity, then begin the first isometric exercise.

When you perform an isometric exercise never hold your breath. Always breathe deeply and naturally, which will be about 10 full breaths in and out at a rate of about 1 second per full breath.

Perform each exercise for no less than 7 seconds, and no longer than 10. Try not to rest between each exercise for longer than 10 seconds, which should allow enough time to recover while getting into the next position.

Once you have assumed the next isometric exercise angle, perform the exercise in the same way as the previous one, and then perform the third angle isometric exercise in the same way.

With the triple isometric portion of the exercise completed, try to rest for no longer than 10 seconds before performing the isotonic phase.

NOTE: Only change arms to perform the isometric exercise with the other arm when you have exercised one arm both isometrically and isotonically.

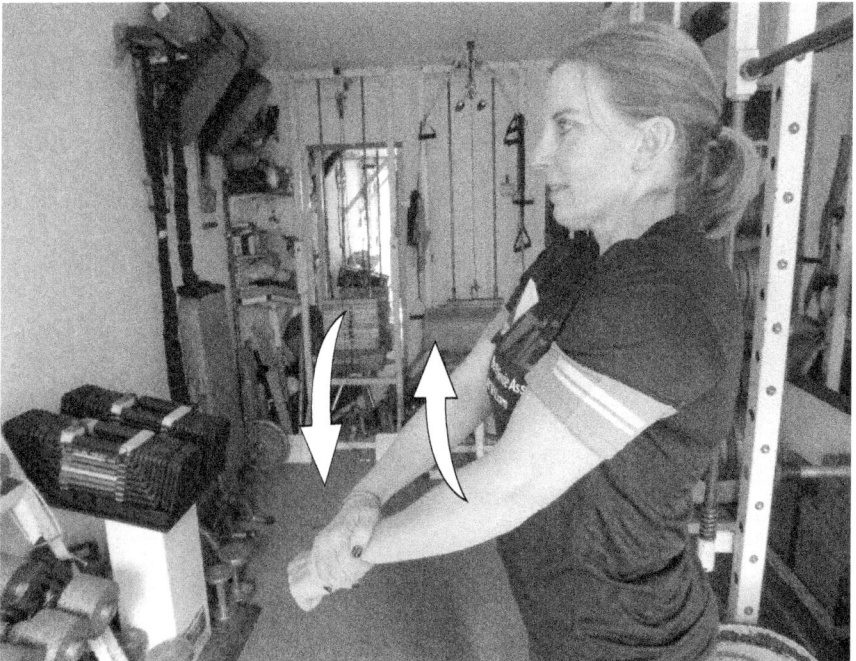

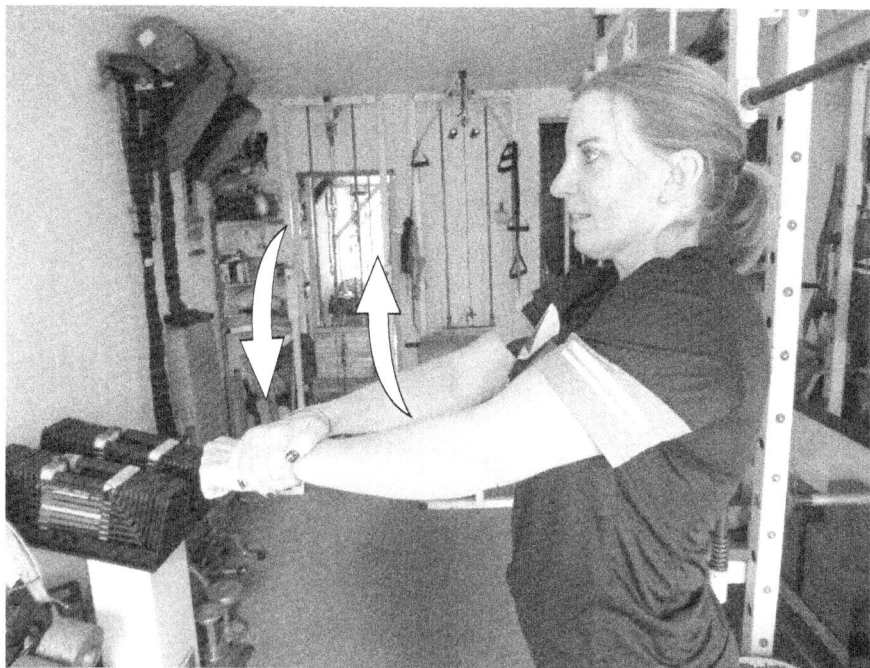

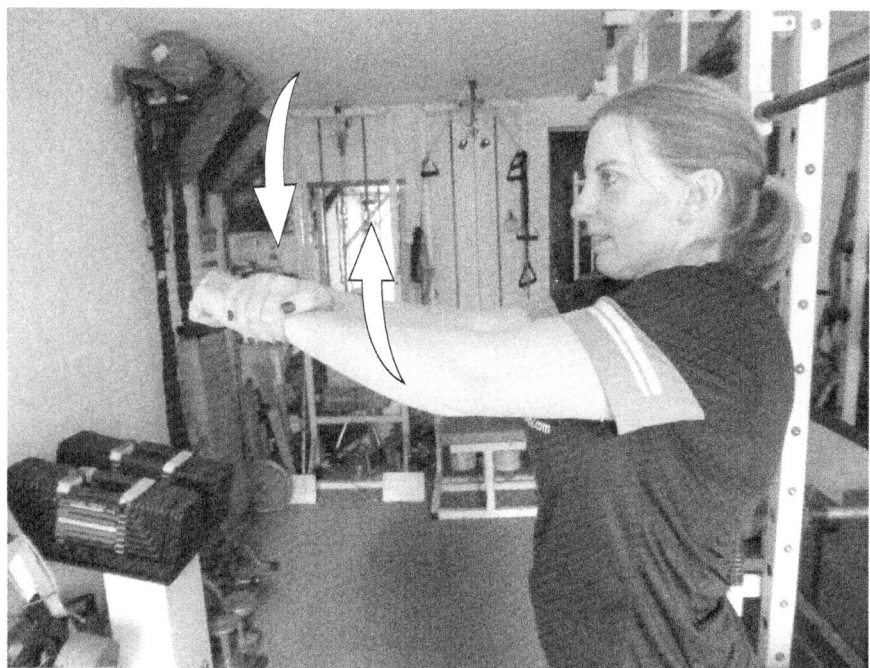

B) Isotonic Front Raise (Left and Right Arm) (Rope / Iso-Bow® / Towel / Hands)

Continuing from the isometric phase with the same arm you have just exercised in three positions. With the arms and hands in the same positions (one fist clenched, and both elbows slightly bent)

Raise the arm with the clenched fist forward and upwards using the front deltoid muscles, and the arm with the open hand serving as the resistance.

The exercise should be performed in super-slow style with each portion of the exercise (eccentric and concentric) taking between 10 and 12 seconds to complete. This makes it extremely challenging by any standards.

Never hold your breath, and a suggested method of breathing during super-slow repetitions is to breathe in and out one full breath for each second of elapsed time.

Aim to perform one set of three repetitions, but do not be surprised if you can only manage one repetition at super-slow speed. If this is your limit, even only one repetition performed at super-slow speed will deliver all the results you desire.

Do not sacrifice good exercise style and true super-slow speed in exchange for a greater number of repetitions at a faster speed.

You will gradually increase the number of repetitions you can perform by following the science and adhering to a strict exercise style and good technique.

NOTE: Only change arms to perform the isometric exercise with the other arm when you have exercised one arm both isometrically and isotonically.

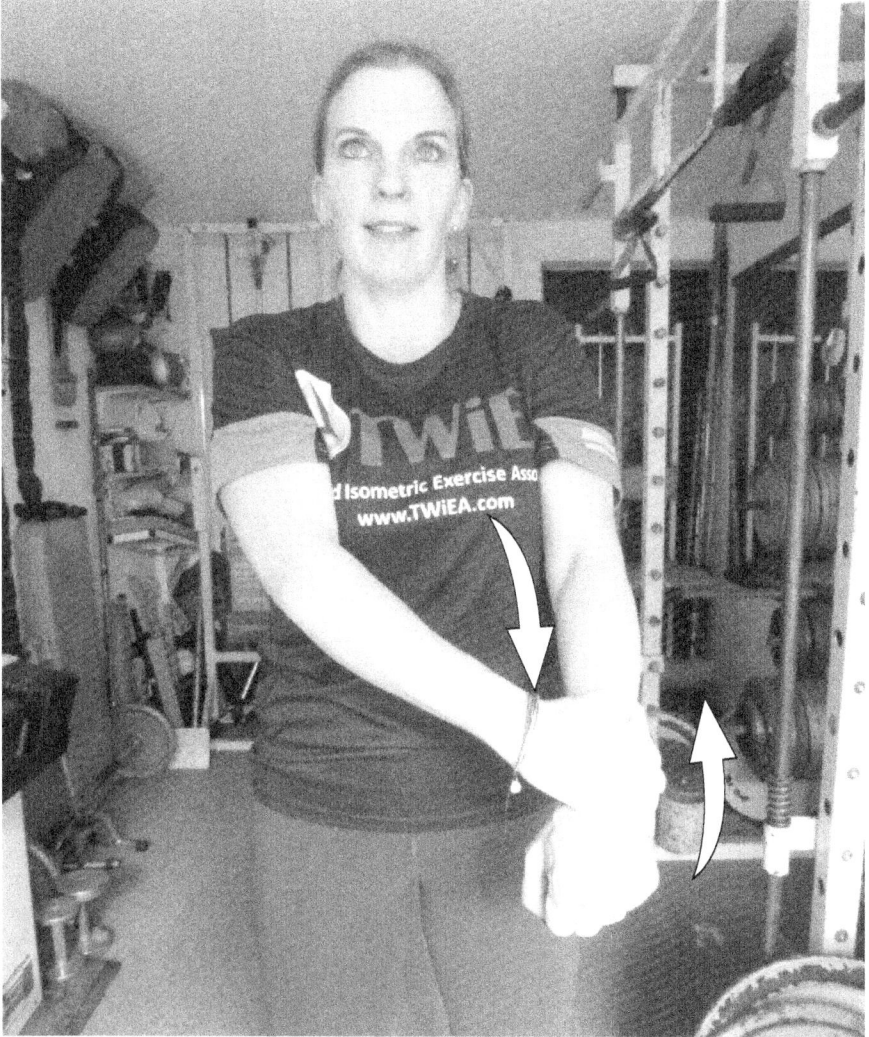

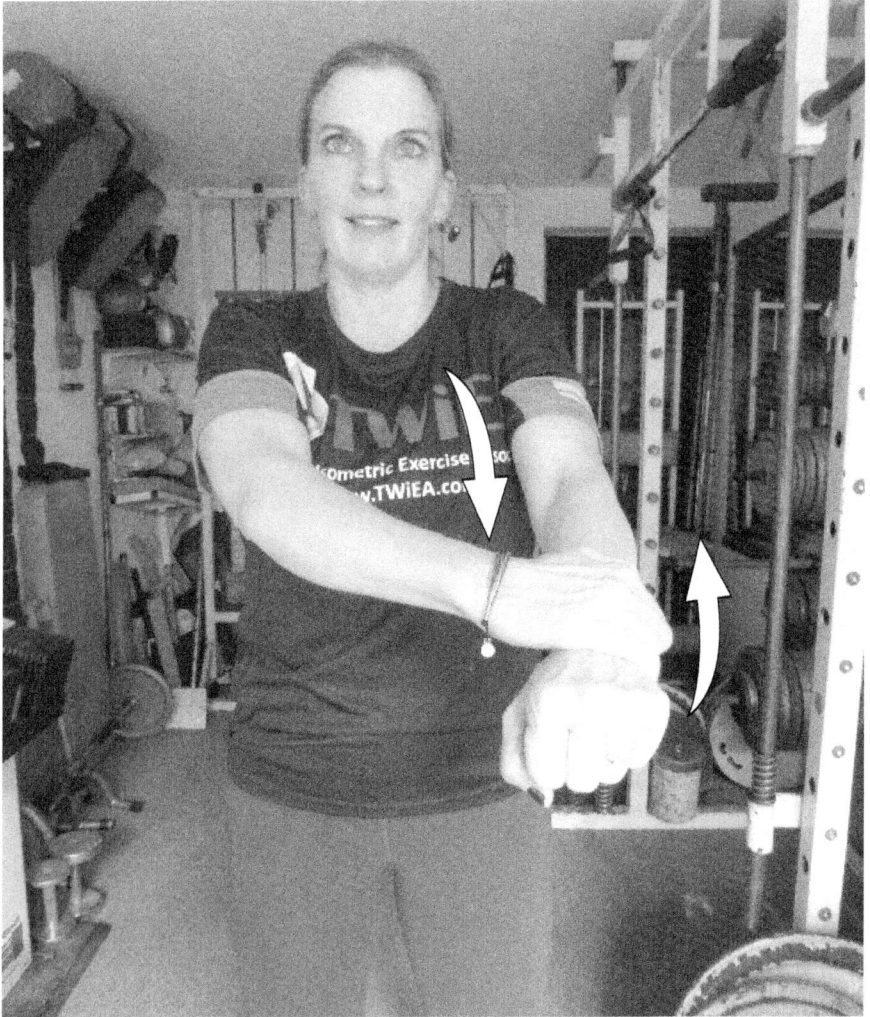

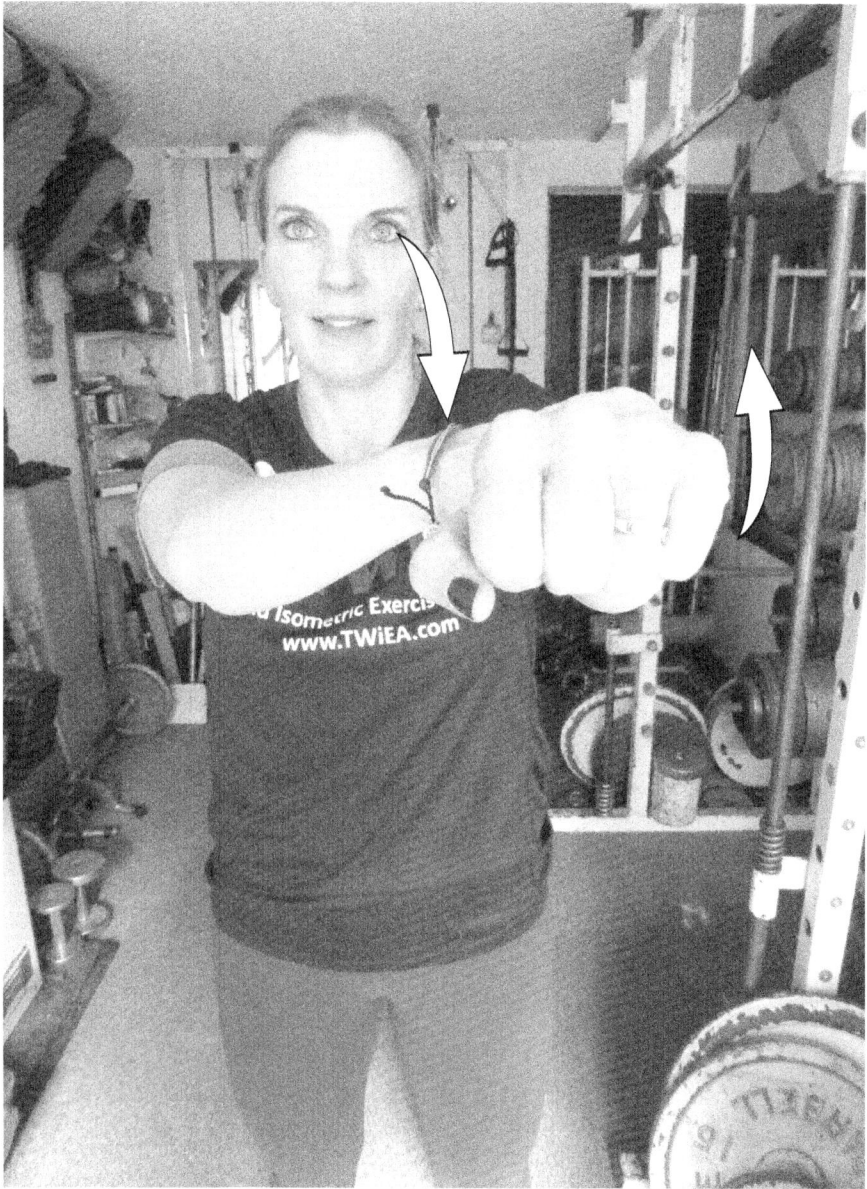

MUM™ Course – 3rd Month Onwards

Begin Bi-Monthly Rotation and Revert Back to Month 1 After Every Second Month has been Completed

For month three, you to go back to month one and repeat the exercises. However, if you have been following the course faithfully through months one and two, then you will be both fitter and stronger.

Therefore, you will be performing the new phase of repeating month one with slightly more effort and intensity than when you began.

Similarly, when you have completed the repeated phase of month one exercises again, then shift into performing the exercises in month two again.

From this point onwards, since this workout is not so intense that it places a strain on your ability to recover and make you retain weight etc., the bi-monthly rotation of these workout plans can be repeated almost indefinitely.

However, once you are familiar with both the process and with a wider variety of exercises, then you experiment by replacing some with new ones.

Chapter 9. Conclusion

We hope that you have found this book both interesting and informative, and I hope that you have gained something from the story of my rather bumpy life journey. I assume that since you read this book that you are a woman who is either facing or going through menopause. Therefore, we wish you well on your journey and hope that we have been able to provide you with several practical solutions you can use to help you.

My journey through menopause is almost over, and at times it has been extremely challenging, despite me having genuinely employed all of the practical solutions in this book. It can be just a fact that some days are better than others. However, all days were significantly better than they would have been if I had not deliberately employed a strategy of positive action to minimise the overall impact of menopause.

Menopause not only impacts a woman physically and emotionally, but it can also significantly impact her relationship with her lifemate if she has one. The myriad of effects menopause brings with it in its wake are both considerable, embarrassing, and extremely frustrating.

For those women who are already experiencing some, or all, of the effects of menopause, all that I can say to them is that I feel your pain because I know exactly what you are dealing with. There are even times when I am thoroughly embarrassed as a female because of the intimate physical failings I have and am still experiencing as a woman with a husband.

I like to be open and honest about these things, so I admit that menopause has meant that I now have to deal with many intimate female issues that were never a problem before menopause. I admit, and joke, that my female parts, or as my husband also jokes with me in calling them "my lady bits in my nether regions" do not function as they previously did. Menopause has meant that my intimate lady parts are now even dryer than the Atacama Desert, and that is saying something profound because the Atacama Desert in South America is officially the driest nonpolar desert in the world. So, forget the Atacama Desert, because there is now a new place that is officially dryer than that!

The problem is that until you experience something like this for yourself, then it can be extremely hard to truly comprehend. Thankfully, aside from me still dealing with problems like this and the most practical solutions I can find to address them, overall, physically at least, my exercise and nutrition approach to dealing with menopause has proven to be a winner for me, my twin sister, and many other friends in similar positions. I have come a long way in my life journey, and in many ways, I have achieved a lot. If nothing else, going from being between 40 and 50 lbs overweight, making me obese for my height, isometric exercise combined with a plant-based diet has worked wonders. The picture on the left is of me before I began my journey, and the one on the following page is at its peak.

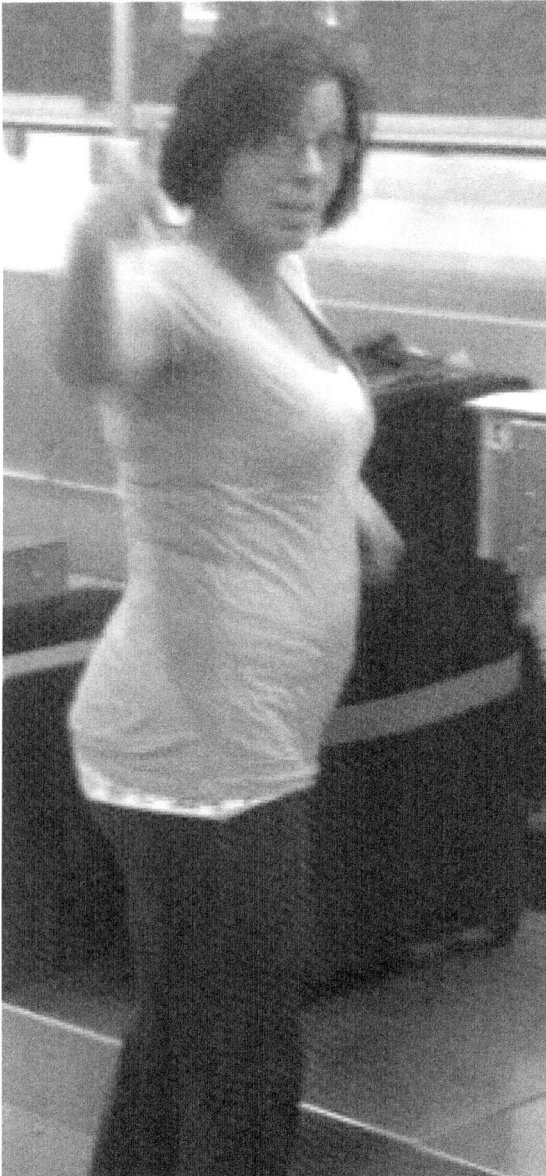

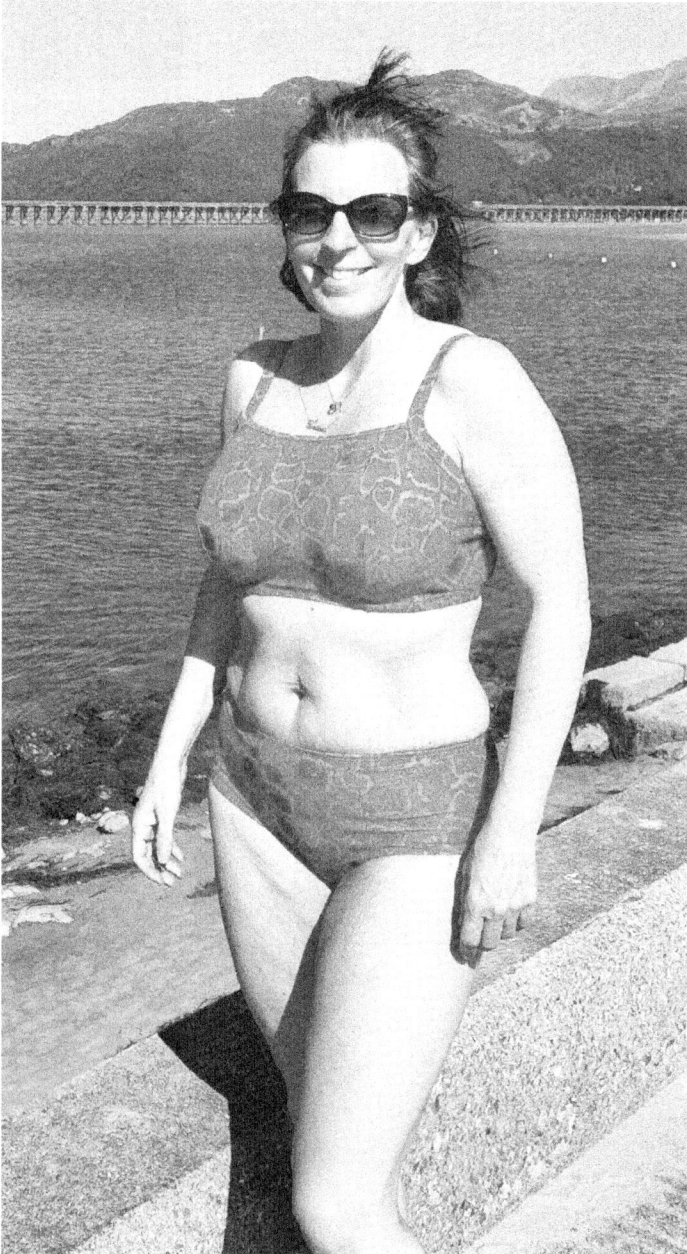

This is me at 51 years old and mid-menopause, in July 2021, in Barmouth, Wales, after performing the Muscle Up for Menopause workout for three months.

Have faith in both isometric exercise and a plant-based diet because they are both scientifically proven to work and deliver many positive health and fitness-related benefits. One of the key factors in my success in using the isometric system for brief exercise sessions has been consistency. Therefore, do not miss an exercise session. Furthermore, you have no excuse to miss a session because everyone, even on their busiest day can find 70 seconds of consecutive exercise time to spare. There are simply no excuses that you cannot exercise this way regularly.

Since I am now an isometric and TRISOmetric™ exercise instructor trainer as part of TWiEA (The World Isometric Exercise Association) I can be contacted via their website at www.TWiEA.com or via my website at www.HelenRenee.com if you have any questions that I might be able to help with. We wish you well and success in all things on your journey through life, and menopause.

What is TWiEA™?

For more information and member's online video resources for TWiEA members, visit www.TWiEA.com. TWiEA™ is the acronym for The World Isometric Exercise Association which is the governing body for all types of isometric exercise. Its mission is to help set and maintain standards of excellence in teaching and promoting all types of isometric exercise. TWiEA™ seeks to ensure that scientifically proven isometric exercise techniques are taught as part of an integrated overall approach to the total-body exercise solutions provided by fitness professionals. This creates a much higher probability that busy clients facing real-life time-crunches can maintain an effective exercise program. Isometric exercise is every bit as effective at building muscle and strength as other traditional forms of resistance training. It is also both a time and money-saving exercise solution that almost anyone can perform without any special equipment.

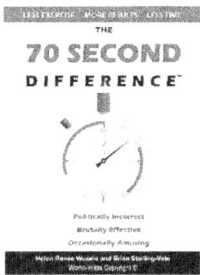

The 70 Second Difference™ - The Politically Incorrect, Occasionally Amusing, and Brutally Effective Guide to Strength, Fitness and Better Health

This book has been approved by **TWiEA** – The World Isometric Exercise Association (www.TWiEA.com).

This is a science-based no-nonsense guide that tells it straight about the most efficient ways to exercise, build muscle, get strong, and how deliberate lifestyle and dietary choices affect you. Lack of time is the main reason why most people don't exercise, however, just 70 seconds a day of focussed science-based exercise can solve the problem. Recommended equipment: 2 x Iso-Bows®

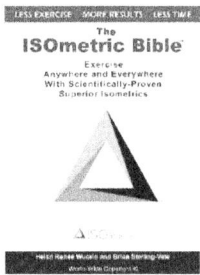

The ISOmetric Bible™ - Exercise Anywhere with Scientifically Proven Isometrics

This book has been approved by **TWiEA** – The World Isometric Exercise Association (www.TWiEA.com).

The ISOmetric Bible™ is a complete, practical, scientific, and user-friendly book. Isometric exercise is proven by science to grow muscle and strength faster and more efficiently than any other exercise system. However, it is also one of the most misunderstood forms of exercise, even by some professionals. No special equipment is needed to get a great total-body workout and this book shows you how to use easy to find everyday objects such as walking poles, broom handles, rope, and towels to exercise with. Recommended equipment: 2 x Iso-Bows®, some climbing rope, and a towel.

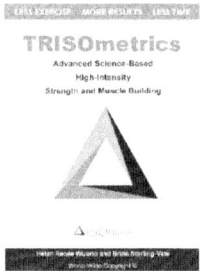

TRISOmetrics™ - Advanced Science-Based High-Intensity Strength and Muscle Building

This book has been approved by **TWiEA** – The World Isometric Exercise Association (www.TWiEA.com).

259

TRISOmetrics™ is an advanced, science-based high-intensity exercise system that combines 3 scientifically proven exercise techniques into a powerful new exercise system. It can be performed with or without equipment either at home or when travelling, or it can be used as part of a gym-based exercise routine. The system is ideal for people who do not confuse activity with accomplishment. Suggested equipment: 2 x Iso-Bows®, climbing rope and a towel. It can also be performed with the Bullworker®, Steel Bow®, and with all gym-based exercise equipment.

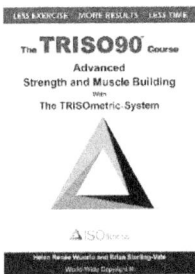

The TRISO90™ Course – Advanced Strength and Muscle Building with The TRISOmetrics™ System

This book has been approved by **TWiEA** – The World Isometric Exercise Association (www.TWiEA.com).

The TRISO90™ Course is a 500+ page 90-day/12-week step-by-step highly advanced bodybuilding/shaping and strength-training exercise course based on the TRISOmetrics™ exercise system. The system consists of three proven science-based exercise principles which when combined, form this highly advanced high-intensity exercise technique, with or without equipment. Suggested equipment: 2 x Iso-Bows®, dipping handles, some climbing rope, and a towel.

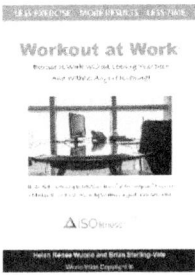

Workout at Work™ - Exercise at Work Without Anyone Even Knowing What You're Doing!

This book has been approved by **TWiEA** – The World Isometric Exercise Association (www.TWiEA.com).

Time is the #1 reason why people do not exercise. The average person spends over 10 years of their life at a desk! With proven isometric exercise, you can exercise effectively at work without ever leaving your desk. Perform just one simple 7-second high-intensity exercise every 30 minutes, and at the end of a 9-hour working day, you will have completed a powerful total-body 18-20 exercise. Your boss will not complain either because in exchange for just 126 seconds of time off work you will be up to 30% more efficient at your job. Recommended equipment: 2 x Iso-Bows®

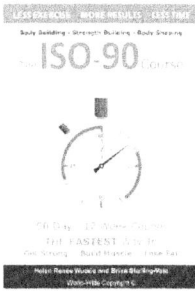

The ISO90™ Course – The 12-Week/90-Day Shape-up and Get Strong Course

This book has been approved by **TWiEA** – The World Isometric Exercise Association (www.TWiEA.com).

The ISO90™ Course is a complete step-by-step 90-day/12-week isometric body shaping, bodybuilding, and strength building course ideal for both beginners and advanced trainers. Your natural Adaptive Response™ mechanism means that whatever intensity you apply at whatever level you are, gives everyone roughly the same percentage of improvement. Required equipment: 2 x Iso-Bows® available on Amazon or from Bullworker.com

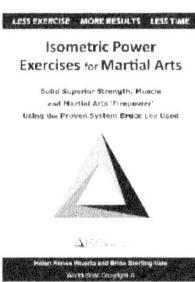

Isometric Power Exercises for Martial Arts™ - Build Superior Strength, Muscle and Martial Arts 'Firepower' Using the Proven System Bruce Lee Used

This book has been approved by **TWiEA** – The World Isometric Exercise Association (www.TWiEA.com).

Isometric exercise has been part of almost every system of martial arts for thousands of years. The great Bruce Lee also loved isometric exercise. This book is a valuable resource of practical isometric exercises to build serious strength, muscle, and martial arts firepower. The author is a leading authority on isometric exercise, has practised martial arts for almost 50-years and is a WKA 8th Degree Black Belt and a recipient of a WKA Lifetime Achievement Award.

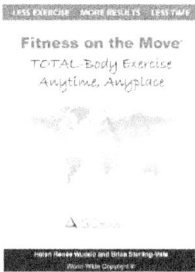

Fitness on the Move™ - Enjoy Gym-Quality Workout Sessions ANYWHERE!

This book has been approved by **TWiEA** – The World Isometric Exercise Association (www.TWiEA.com).

261

This book lists practical exercises that can be performed while travelling as passengers in cars, on trains, in airline seats, on mountainsides, and beaches etc. A total-body workout can be performed in the smallest space humanly possible thanks to our Zero Footprint Workout™ concept. If there is enough space to either sit down and/or stand upright, then you can perform exercise! Required/suggested equipment: 2 x Iso-Bows®

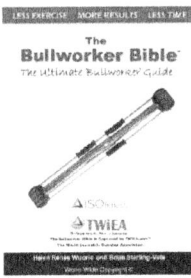

The Bullworker Bible™ The Ultimate Science-Based Guide to The Classic Personal Multi-Gym

This book has been approved by **TWiEA** – The World Isometric Exercise Association (www.TWiEA.com) and the makers of The Bullworker.

The Bullworker Bible™ is THE resource guide for all Bullworker® users and is the companion book to The Bullworker 90™ Course. It is complete, science-based, and user-friendly showing how it should be used to deliver maximum results with information about repetition-compression and speed, breathing, how the laws of physics apply, and correct biomechanics. It is also essential for users of the Steel Bow®, the X5, Bully Extreme, ISO 7x, and the X7. Required: Bullworker® Classic, or similar. Recommended additional equipment: Steel Bow®, 2 x Iso-Bows®.

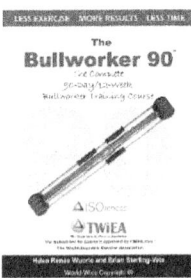

The Bullworker 90™ Course – The Ultimate Science-Based 12-Week/90-Day Get strong and Grow Muscle Course Using the Classic Personal Multi-Gym

This book has been approved by **TWiEA** – The World Isometric Exercise Association (www.TWiEA.com) and the makers of The Bullworker.

The Bullworker 90™ Course is a 90-day/12-week step-by-step course for all Bullworker® users and is the companion book to The Bullworker Bible™. Each week has a detailed note section, so you know exactly what to do and when to do it. It can be used with the Bullworker® Classic, the Steel Bow®, the X5, the Bully Extreme, the ISO 7x, and the X7. The course contains alternative/extra exercises using the Iso-Bow® and the Bow Extension®. Required equipment: Bullworker® Classic, or similar.

Recommended equipment: Steel Bow®, Bow Extension® kit, 2 x Iso-Bows®.

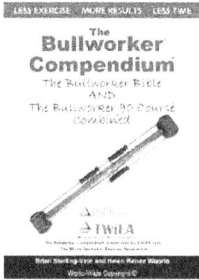

The Bullworker Compendium™ - The Bullworker Bible™ and The Bullworker90™ Course Combined

This book has been approved by **TWiEA** – The World Isometric Exercise Association (www.TWiEA.com) and the makers of The Bullworker.

The Bullworker Compendium™ is the combination of both The Bullworker Bible™ and The Bullworker 90™ Course in a single huge book.   To save printing costs the only thing we have eliminated are duplicated sections, everything else remains the same.   This way we can offer both books in one for less than the combined price of the two other books.   It starts with The Bullworker Bible™ and progresses seamlessly into The Bullworker 90™ Course.

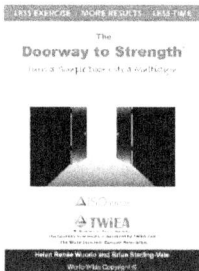

The Doorway to Strength™ - Turn a Door into a Strength-Building Multigym

This book has been approved by **TWiEA** – The World Isometric Exercise Association (www.TWiEA.com).

The Doorway to Strength™ shows how a simple door, doorway, and doorframe can be used to create a multi-gym of exercises using the amazing Iso-Bow® exerciser. It demonstrates how to perform a host of powerful and effective isometric exercises such as the door leg press and shoulder power push, together with many other exercises to work all the major body parts. Required: 2 x Iso-Bows®, a solid door and frame, and a door wedge/stop.

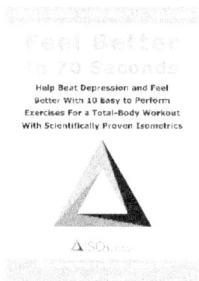

Feel Better In 70 Seconds™
Help Beat Depression and Feel Better With 10 Easy to Perform Exercises For a Total-Body Workout With Scientifically Proven Isometrics

This book has been approved by TWiEA – The World Isometric Exercise Association (www.TWiEA.com). Isolation, depression loneliness, anxiety, and stress are just a few of the serious mental health issues that millions of us can suffer from during our life. Research shows that exercise can help to beat depression and that exercise can be equal to or often better than medication. How can you exercise if you have little or no money, space, motivation, and no idea about exercise? The 70 Second Difference™ is a protocol based upon the premise that 70 seconds of consecutive exercise is needed to perform a 10-exercise total-body workout routine using the scientifically proven isometric exercise system. There is no exercise system we know of that is faster, more effective, and easier to perform.

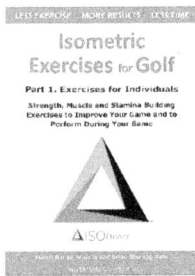

Isometric Exercises for Golf™ Part 1. Exercises for Individuals

This book has been approved by **TWiEA** – The World Isometric Exercise Association (www.TWiEA.com).

There is no such thing as a quick game of golf which means there is not always enough spare time to exercise in a gym as well. A series of advanced 7 to 10-second isometric exercises either while you play or practice is the answer. Perform just one isometric exercise at each hole and at the end of an 18-hole game you have completed a powerful total-body workout. The average golf club is a perfect Improvised Isometric Exercise Device or IIED, so you are carrying your go-anywhere multi-gym everywhere you play. Part 1. is a resource guide of isometric exercises that can be performed as an individual. Note: The exercises in this book are either the same or similar to those in our books: Nordic Walking or Trekking Pole. The Isometric Exercises for Golf book 1 contains some special exercises designed to increase the strength and power of your golf swing.

Isometric Exercises for Golf™ Part 2. Exercises for Partner-Pairs

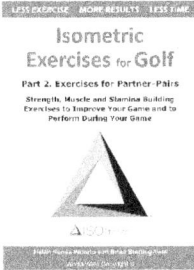

This book has been approved by TWiEA – The World Isometric Exercise Association (www.TWiEA.com).

This is the companion to Book 1 and is focussed on exercises that are best performed in partnered pairs, with a friend during a break, a game, or during practice sessions.

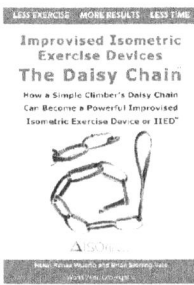

Improvised Isometric Exercise Devices - The Daisy Chain - How a Simple Climber's Daisy Chain Can Become a Powerful Improvised Isometric Exercise Device or IIED

This book has been approved by TWiEA – The World Isometric Exercise Association (www.TWiEA.com).

Improvised Isometric Exercise Devices or IIEDs come in all shapes and sizes and are only limited by your imagination and knowledge of good biomechanics. Basic climbing equipment can also become extremely powerful IIEDs and is both expensive and non-proprietary. One of the most effective is the versatile daisy chain. This is a valuable resource listing improvised and practical isometric exercises that can be performed as well as how to safely extend the device.

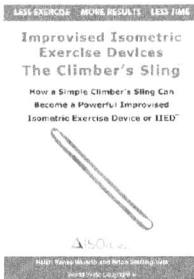

Improvised Isometric Exercise Devices - The Climber's Sling - How a Simple Climber's Sling Can Become a Powerful Improvised Isometric Exercise Device or IIED

This book has been approved by TWiEA – The World Isometric Exercise Association (www.TWiEA.com).

Improvised Isometric Exercise Devices or IIEDs come in all shapes and sizes and are only limited by your imagination and knowledge of good biomechanics. Basic climbing equipment can also become extremely powerful IIEDs and is both expensive and non-proprietary. One of the most effective is the versatile Climber's sling. This is a valuable resource listing improvised and practical isometric exercises that can be performed as well as how to safely extend the device.

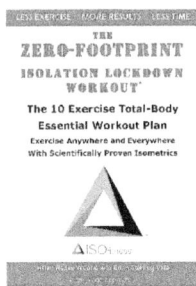

The Zero-Footprint Isolation Lockdown Workout
The 10 Exercise Total-Body Essential Workout Plan
Exercise Anywhere and Everywhere With Scientifically Proven Isometrics

This book has been approved by TWiEA – The World Isometric Exercise Association (www.TWiEA.com).

In 2020, the world changed forever due to the COVID-19 global pandemic and gyms are typically some of the unhealthiest of places when it comes to virus and disease transmissions. Millions of people who love to exercise were suddenly forced to learn how to exercise at home, sometimes in very confined spaces. The Zero-Footprint Isolation Lockdown Workout™ delivers the 10-essential total-body isometric exercises that can be performed in the smallest of spaces. If you can stand and sit, then you can perform a powerful workout routine in as little as 70 seconds a day! NOTE: This is a variation of The 70 Second Difference™ workout.

The Sixty Second ASS Workout™ - The Ultimate 60-Second Workout to Shape, Tone, Lift and Give You the Backside You've Always Wanted

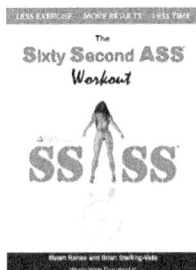

This book has been approved by **TWiEA** – The World Isometric Exercise Association (www.TWiEA.com).

The Sixty Second ASS Workout™, or SSASS™ workout, is the fastest and most effective "ass" workout ever devised. Scientifically proven advanced isometric exercises deliver a no-nonsense time-efficient workout that does everything you need to make your backside tight, firm, shapely and strong. No more time-wasting workouts where you twist, shake, wiggle around that might be fun but never deliver the results you want. Everyone has 60 seconds to spare, even on the busiest day, so, you are just 60 seconds a day from having a great ass. Required Equipment: 2 x Iso-Bows.

Isometric Exercises for Nordic Walking and Trekking™ - Part 1. Exercises for Individuals

This book has been approved by **TWiEA** – The World Isometric Exercise Association (www.TWiEA.com).

More Nordic Walkers and Trekkers than ever before perform proven gym-quality total-body isometric exercise routines during scheduled walk breaks in almost any location using their walking/trekking poles as an IIED or Improvised Isometric Exercise Device. Book 1. is an resource guide of isometric exercises that can be performed as an individual, either outdoors or at home. Note: The exercises in this book are either the same or similar to those in our other books using a golf club. However, the Isometric Exercises for Golf book 1 contains some special exercises designed to increase the strength and power of your golf swing.

Isometric Exercises for Nordic Walking and Trekking™ - Part 2. Exercises for Walk Partner-Pairs

This book has been approved by **TWiEA** – The World Isometric Exercise Association (www.TWiEA.com).

This is the companion to Book 1 and is focussed on exercises that are best performed as a partner-pair, with a friend during a walking break anywhere.

Being American Married to a Brit™ - An Amusing Guide for Anglo-American Couples Divided by a Common Language and Culture

When I first started dating my British man, I never gave a second thought about differences in language

267

and culture. Why would I? After all, we Americans speak English, or do we...? As dating quickly turned into an engagement and then being married to my British gentleman, our common language and culture was a quirky, eye-opening, and highly amusing roller-coaster ride. At times during the most basic everyday conversations, I would be listening to his words with glazed eyes, wondering what on earth he was saying. It was as if we were both speaking a different language. I decided to write this book and dedicate it to all transatlantic couples who will regularly find themselves completely divided and confused by their common language and culture.

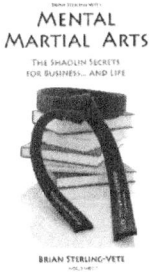

Mental Martial Arts™ - intellectual Life and Business Combat Skills

Brian Sterling-Vete's Mental Martial Arts is a system of intellectual life-combat skills using the tactics and principles of the physical martial arts. All interaction in life, business, and when communicating with others is an exchange of energy, power, and influence. Each party is always exerting maximum influence over the other to gain the outcome they prefer. The more powerful and persuasive will usually win unless the apparently weaker person is trained in the Mental Martial Arts. You can learn how to verbally, intellectually, and emotionally guide, channel, and redirect the energy of others, even powerful people, and large organisations to more frequently achieve the outcomes that you desire in life and business. It contains a section about how to handle a potentially hostile news media in a crisis from experience gained over a decade with BBC TV News and a lifetime in martial arts to help you and your organisation stay Media Safe.

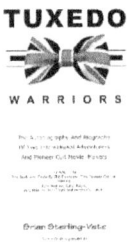

Tuxedo Warriors™

Tuxedo Warriors is the companion book to both The Tuxedo Warrior book and movie. These books are the biography and autobiography of the iconic cult author, composer, moviemaker Cliff Twemlow. The original book ended at the beginning of what has been called by many the Golden Age of Video Cinematography which Cliff inspired. Tuxedo Warriors continues the story from where his original book finishes, and it is the most complete biography of Cliff Twemlow ever written. It is also the autobiography of Brian Sterling-Vete who played a central role in this unique, entertaining, and true story of their adventures as guerrilla moviemakers.

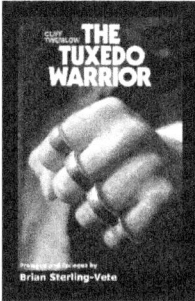

The Tuxedo Warrior™ by Cliff Twemlow – Prologue and epilogue by Brian Sterling-Vete.

There are many ways in which a Doorman can gain respect. Numerous methods were applied to the principal. In my profession, every available technique must be utilised, depending on the situation and circumstances. Would-be transgressors either move off the premises and quietly acknowledge your diplomatic approach. Or, the other alternative whereby physical persuasion must be exercised, which either quells their pugilistic desires or it triggers their aggressive instincts, turning the whole incident into a bloody and violent encounter. 'The Tuxedo Warrior,' pulls no punches in its brawling, savage, colourful, and entertaining exposure of society's nightlife activities.

The above is the original text from the rear cover of Cliff's book. Where his book finishes, my book *Tuxedo Warriors* begins to complete Cliff's colourful life story. I am honoured to be friends with Cliff's eldest son, Barry, and sincerely thank him for enabling this book and the others his father wrote to be re-published.

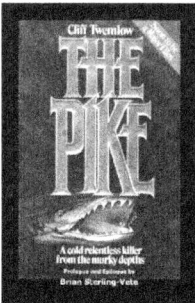

The Pike™ by Cliff Twemlow – Prologue and epilogue by Brian Sterling-Vete.

ITS FIRST VICTIMS - A screeching swan… A fisherman overboard… A drunken woman…

One by one, the mysterious killer in Lake Windermere claims its terrified victims. Tearing off limbs with its monstrous teeth, horribly mutilating bodies. Fear sweeps the peaceful holiday resort when experts identify the creature as a giant pike…. A hellish creature with the strength to rupture boats, and the anger to attack them. But for some, the terror becomes a bonanza—the traders who cater to the gathering crowds of ghouls on the shore. And they will do anything to stop divers from finding the creature. Meanwhile the ripples of bloodshed widen…. The Pike.

The above is the original text from the rear cover of Cliff's book which was to become a movie in the early 1980s starring Joan Collins.

The Beast of Kane™ by Cliff Twemlow – Prologue and epilogue by Brian Sterling-Vete.

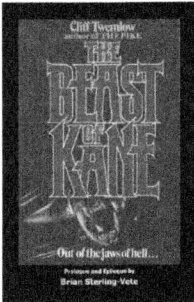

When the Gordon Family open their door to a stray Elkhound, they unwittingly welcome in the forces of evil. For, according to the local priest, the huge dog is Satan himself, fulfilling an ancient prophecy. But no one will believe this warning… Even when sheep – and wolves – are mysteriously slaughtered. Even when frenzied pets turn on their owners. Even when Emily Forrest is savagely eaten alive – the first of many human victims. As winter tightens its icy grip on the remote town of Kane, its unprotected people must face an unearthly terror.

The above is the original text from the rear cover of Cliff's book. This was the first of Cliff's books to be accepted by Hammer Film Studios to become a big-screen horror movie, along with Cliff's other book, The Pike.

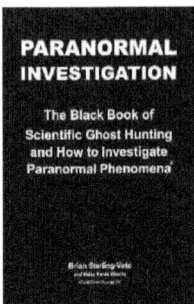

Paranormal Investigation - The Black Book of Scientific Ghost Hunting and How to Investigate Paranormal Phenomena™

This book is ideal for those who are new to paranormal investigation, and for more experienced investigators who want to learn more about how to apply a more scientific approach. It contains a special scientific critical path graphic page to work from when devising ghost hunting experiments and to help train team members. There is a step-by-step guide to a complete paranormal investigation and vital information about how to protect yourself from malevolent paranormal entities that can attack you. It also contains ideas for potentially paranormally active and 'haunted' locations and several accounts of previously untold paranormal events including the remarkable Redwood Falls Minnesota UFO sighting.

The Haunting of Lilford Hall™ - The Birthplace of the United States as a Nation Haunted by the Man Behind The Pilgrim Fathers

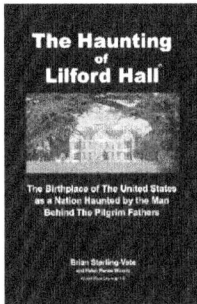

The Haunting of Lilford Hall is one of the most baffling cases ever recorded of paranormal activity experienced simultaneously by multiple people. Between 2012 and 2013, a team of 13 people produced a historical TV documentary about the life of Robert Browne, the man who was behind The Pilgrim Fathers sailing on The Mayflower to settle the first civilian colony on the American continent. Without Robert Browne, there may never have been the United States of America, at least not as we know it today. They experienced doors that refused to stay closed, they had debris thrown at them, they had a door silently ripped away from the hinges and doorframe while they were in the next room. There were even several recorded multi-witness apparitions of a man fitting Robert Browne's recorded description. It is believed by many that the ghost of Robert Browne, the "Grandfather" of the United States as a nation, still haunts Lilford Hall.

- Robert Browne was the man who first separated the church from the state which is the underpinning of the United States.
- Robert Browne's words are written into the U.S. constitution.
- Robert Browne's direct descendent officially fired the first shot in the American war of independence.
- Robert Browne's beloved Lilford Hall estate home to President George Washington's mother & President Quincy Adams' family.

www.MajorVision.com - www.TWiEA.com

Printed in Great Britain
by Amazon